IN
MYSTERIOUS
WAYS

IN MYSTERIOUS WAYS

❀

The Death and Life of a Parish Priest

Paul Wilkes

GROVE PRESS
New York

First published in 1990 in New York by Random House, Inc.

A portion of this work was originally published in different form in *The New Yorker.*

Grateful acknowledgment is made to the Macmillan Publishing Company and Editions Plon for permission to reprint excerpts from *The Diary of a Country Priest* by George Bernanos, translated from the French by Pamela Morris. Copyright © 1933 by the Macmillan Company. Copyright renewed 1965 by Macmillan Publishing Company. Rights throughout the world excluding the United States are controlled by Editions Plon. Reprinted by permission of Macmillan Publishing Company and Editions Plon.

Published simultaneously in Canada
Printed in the United States of America

FIRST GROVE PRESS EDITION

Library of Congress Cataloging-in-Publication Data
Wilkes, Paul, 1938–
    In mysterious ways : the death and life of a parish priest / Paul Wilkes.
    p. cm.
    Originally published: 1st ed. New York : Random House, 1990.
    ISBN 0-8021-3851-9
    1. Greer, Joseph. 2. Catholic Church—United States—Clergy—
Biography. 3. Cancer—Patients—United States—Biography. I. Title.

BX4705.G6188 W55 2001
282'.092—dc21
[B]   2001042487

Grove Press
841 Broadway
New York, NY 10003

01 02 03 04   10 9 8 7 6 5 4 3 2 1

For Tracy

ACKNOWLEDGMENTS

Two fine editors made this book possible. Bob Gottlieb at *The New Yorker* saw in Father Greer a way to tell not only of a man but of a unique time in the life of America's Catholic Church. Sam Vaughan at Random House allowed me to tell the fuller story of Father Greer's work and harrowing bone marrow transplant. Writers are not often blessed to have two such men to work with. They were insightful and encouraging. Who could ask for more?

Sara Lippincott at *The New Yorker* put an enormous amount of time and attention into shaping my original profile, and Olga Tarnowski at Random House went steps further, first to make my words say what I wanted them to, and then to shepherd those words into print. Lynn Anderson deftly copy-edited the final manuscript.

The Archdiocese of Boston was most helpful in my original search for a "country priest," and special thanks go to Father Ernest Serino for recommending Father Greer.

Dr. Jane Desforges at the New England Medical Center was unfailingly available to me and allowed me to see modern medicine up close. She and her colleagues in hematology patiently answered the questions of a man whose knowledge of science was pathetically limited.

During my many days and nights at St. Patrick's rectory, Janet Hamilton, Anna Caruso, and Dolly Peters were most kind and helpful.

A special thanks goes to Alison Bond, my agent. In full season and fallow, she always believed.

Father Bernard Bonowitz, OCSO, a Trappist monk at St. Joseph's Abbey in Spencer, Massachusetts, was my first reader. His amazing breadth of knowledge greatly helped me.

He comforts us in all our afflictions and thus enables us to comfort those who are in trouble, with the same consolation we have received from Him. As we have shared much in the suffering of Christ, so through Christ do we share abundantly in His consolation.

2 Corinthians 1:3

I owe a great debt to Father Joseph Greer. He allowed me to view firsthand the many functions, duties, and rituals of a parish priest. He permitted me to be present for much of his medical treatment and then assisted me in reconstructing what he had gone through during the worst days of his illness and hospitalizations.

He gave me access to his inner self. He stayed the course.

INTRODUCTION

I met Father Joseph Greer under rather odd circumstances. In 1987 I wrote to the Archdiocese of Boston asking to be put into contact with any priests who were suffering from a life-threatening illness and faced imminent death. My idea was to do a documentary film and a book—a modern-day corollary to Georges Bernanos's spiritual classic *The Diary of a Country Priest*—following a parish priest as he lived his last days. Bernanos's fictional portrait of a dying priest in a small, obscure French village had always fascinated and troubled me, revealing as it did such towering heroism in the midst of numbing banality.

Unknown to his parishioners, the priest in that remote French village was struggling with his own inner demons as he daily tried to support and foster their fragile faith. How would this be played out in the life of an American priest serving in a parish today?

I wanted to witness how his parishioners, who once had looked to him for strength and certainty, dealt with his progressive weakness. I wanted to follow such a man through this difficult time and to see what his spirituality meant to him as he faced physical decline and imminent death.

At once impelled by the prospects of finding such a modern day Curé d'Ambricourt, but feeling squeamish about the very personal questions I would have to ask, I visited some half-dozen priests in the Boston area. I was hoping to find the right subject; simultaneously I found myself apprehensive of what might eventually transpire if I did.

A Father Greer was recommended to me by Father Ernest Serino, himself a heart attack victim, who had just conducted a parish renewal at Father Greer's church, St. Patrick's, in Natick, a Boston suburb. He knew Father Greer, although not well, and had been impressed with the spirit of the parish during the week of nightly services he had conducted, as well as with the rectitude of its pastor. "Joe Greer's always been known as a good administrator," Father Serino said, "a solid priest, though not really distinguished. But he's had a blood cancer. I think it's had a profound effect on him. Go talk to him. I don't see how he still does it. The drain on him these days is brutal; it's what made me resign from day-to-day parish work."

When I did go to see Father Greer, I found out in our first meeting that he had been receiving chemotherapy for the past year, and the cancer, a blood disease called multiple myeloma, was responding well to the treatment. He hoped to be told soon, during one of his monthly visits to the New England Medical Center in Boston, that his illness was in total remission. I closed my notebook and told Father Greer that I was happy for him that he had disappointed me with his report of improving health. He would not be my subject.

In the weeks that followed, something about this man, unlike the other priests I had interviewed, remained with me. In the hour we had talked, his milky blue eyes had exhibited everything from a bloodhound's sadness to a leprechaun's mischievous gaiety. I could not remember another face that at one moment appeared so vibrant, alive, and present, then suddenly turned mournful, sad, and distant. His skin would be glowing and then, in an instant, look like crushed, dull parchment. In a church that had seen upheaval over the past few decades, here was a man, I began to sense, who had felt it deeply in his own life.

There was also—and I could describe it to myself in no other way—a basic goodness about him, which seemed to be complemented by a certain toughness. He had a wonderful offhand sense of humor and was straightforward with me, answering any question I put to him. But unlike many individuals a writer interviews, Father Greer did not eagerly volunteer information so as to make his life or person more interesting, complex, compelling, or praiseworthy. I liked him immediately and enormously, and so I arranged to see him again, not knowing exactly why. He was obviously not the priest I was looking for; he did not fit the neat little category I had in mind.

It was at a second and longer meeting with him that I learned more about his illness as well as his priestly calling, his diverse work in five earlier parishes, the struggle to remain a priest during a time when so many of his seminary classmates had left, his duties at St. Patrick's, and his hopes for the people of the parish. I heard nothing of his spirituality; Father Greer was not one to talk of such things directly.

Of the illness: he told me that on Palm Sunday evening the year before he had been in his room when the nagging backache he had been experiencing for the previous few months developed into a searing pain that brought him to his knees. There were also stabbing pains in his bowels and he found he could not void. The pain was so intense he had contorted himself into a fetal position in an attempt to find relief, but no relief had come. He was shaking uncontrollably. He crawled into the bathroom, took a shower, and almost lost consciousness.

Father Greer had always been in excellent physical condition and had been jogging eight or ten miles twice a week, so he tried to shrug off the attack. A day later, walking four blocks from the rectory to the bank, he had to sit down several times and rest on the curb, gasping from pain and fatigue. The day after that, one of his curates found him almost passed out on the rectory stairs. His normally ruddy face was white. Father Greer realized this was more than a fleeting bout of pain.

He spent a few days at Leonard Morse, the local Natick hospital, and then, on the advice of a young cardiologist who had married the daughter of friends, he was admitted to New England Medical Center. Tests were performed under the supervision of Dr. Jane F. Desforges, a leading hematologist at the center, and Father Greer's bone marrow showed a significant buildup of monoclonal protein— an overgrowth of similar cells—which is a classic indication of multiple myeloma. Multiple myeloma is a cancer of the plasma cells found in bone marrow, which normally produces antibodies for the immune system. Because of the proliferation of these unhealthy cells, normal blood cell growth is progressively inhibited.

Even as he told me about his disease and that there was no known cure for it, I could detect no trace of self-pity. There was work to be done at St. Patrick's—this, his new assignment, was foremost in his mind. The physical plant had been sorrily neglected for years and so had the congregation. The people of St. Patrick's had lapsed into a certain complacency, which, Father Greer was quick to say with a knowing but somewhat wan smile, was all too typical in Catholic parishes today.

The work that awaited him constantly presented itself during our conversation as we sat in a simply furnished office off the rectory's first-floor parlor. His custodian reported that a rug had been stolen from the lower church. A woman who was sure she had been poisoned by her landlord's faulty heating system wanted an immediate appointment. Another caller told Father Greer she was not "of the faith" but a Catholic friend was coming from out of town and would he please recite the daily and Sunday Mass schedule. The Metropolitan Boston Transit Authority was not about to pay for the use of the church parking lot its commuters had claimed as their own, and a Natick resident wanted to know why the cardinal had taken the drastic step of ordering it closed. "The cardinal didn't authorize closing the lot, I did," Father Greer replied. "Let's see what happens when a couple hundred cars are dumped on the streets of Natick Monday morning. Maybe that will get the MBTA's attention."

"Some good days and some not so hot," he answered another call, "but basically can't complain; but how about *you?*" immediately turning the conversation from himself. "Hate to put on the Judas shirt, but how about a couple of Celtic tickets for the raffle again this year?"

He was guileless and canny, patient and weary, disappointed and amused.

It was dawning on me that it might be far more interesting to write about a healthy working priest than to seek one who fulfilled my arbitrary "country priest" specifications.

Something else drew me to Father Greer. On the surface he was an interesting man, but I sensed there was much more to him. I wanted to get to know him. And I knew that through him I would also come to better understand the church into which I had been born and of which I had been a member, in varying degrees of earnestness, for most of my life.

On an impulse I abandoned my original project and asked Father Greer if I might spend some time with him, finding out what the life of a parish priest was like these days.

He said I could.

For reasons that will be obvious to the reader, I have protected the privacy of certain people mentioned in the text by changing their names. Such changes are indicated by an asterisk at the first reference to the name.

Part I

I

*The church has a body and a soul; she has to attend to the
needs of her body. A sensible man is not ashamed of eating.*

St. Patrick's, Father Joseph Greer's parish, covers almost four square
miles of the town of Natick and, with eighty-five hundred members,
encompasses one of the larger Catholic communities in suburban
Boston. Its church, which consists of a main sanctuary and a lower
church, seats eleven hundred people. In addition, there is a sixteen-
acre cemetery, a huge elementary school building and adjoining
hall, an eighteen-bedroom convent, and a twenty-seven-room rectory converted from a Civil War–era roadhouse. St. Patrick's, which
was founded in 1860, is for Catholics the mother church of Natick,
having spawned two other churches as the population grew. At one
time being its pastor was considered a dream assignment. For decades the pastor of St. Patrick's had five full-time assistant priests and
commanded, by position if not by birth, the kind of respect customarily reserved for Boston's upper class.

Up until the past twenty years or so, the main and lower churches
of St. Patrick's were often filled beyond their seating capacity at all
but the earliest of Sunday Masses by a legion of loyal Catholics who
would not think of defaulting on their weekly obligation. A full
complement of nuns taught in a school—kindergarten through
eighth grade—whose rooms were crowded with young girls in green

The quotations at the beginning of each chapter and at the conclusion of the book are from
The Diary of a Country Priest by Georges Bernanos.

tartan skirts and crisp white blouses, boys in dark trousers, white shirt, and tie. At one time the enrollment was over eight hundred students. Mealtime at the rectory was a command performance for all priests in residence, regally presided over by the pastor. Three women served, listening attentively for the sound of the bell at the pastor's place at the head of the table, which would indicate some need of the priests was unmet. Fine crystal and china, linen table-cloths and napkins were customary. Within the parish the pastor was looked upon as a grand patriarch and spiritual leader, but his work was primarily administrative. He said a Mass each day, at a time of his own choosing, and apportioned the work of the parish to his assistants. If he officiated at a wedding, funeral, or baptism, it was that of a blood relation or a member of one of Natick's better families. He collected money from his parishioners ardently and consistently and disbursed it without accountability. His word and wishes were unquestioningly obeyed by his priests and his parish-ioners.

But in the years since the Second Vatican Council, which lasted from 1963 to 1965, when Pope John XXIII threw open the windows of an airtight, secure Catholic church, the winds of change have blown harshly over St. Patrick's. Today, Father Greer looks across East Central Street to a closed school building he has no idea how to utilize, and out back to the old parish clubhouse, which has been suggested as a house for the homeless—a seeming anomaly and not a small disconcertion in this well-kept community, until recently inhabited primarily by Italian and Irish immigrants and their de-scendants. The gutters on his rectory are leaking, paint is peeling, the wall covering in his lower church is scaling like the skin of a molting animal. He has two assistants, but because of the decreasing number of available priests, he has been told he will soon lose one of them. As for the kind of deference shown his predecessors, Father Greer, the fifth pastor in St. Patrick's history, can only smile at the memory.

Conversely, the town of Natick itself is booming, thanks to its proximity to Route 128 and Interstate 495, where such high-technology giants as the Digital Equipment Corporation, Data Gen-eral, and Raytheon are situated, and to Route 9, where two sprawling shopping malls are planning to double in size. One-acre zoning,

$500,000 houses, and a rash of condominiums have come to an area once considered little more than a prosaic stop on the commuter line out of Boston.

Earlier, over half the parishioners within the parish's boundaries could be expected at St. Patrick's each Sunday; now attendance has dropped to a quarter.

And the skyrocketing real estate prices are driving out, among others, the Catholic sons and daughters of older Natick residents; in their place come those called DINKs, couples with Double Income, No Kids. Most of these newcomers either are not Catholic or show little interest in practicing their faith.

Father Greer is fifty-five years old and has black hair that ascends to a small wave before being slicked back from his face. The face itself is handsome, strong, and ruddy, relatively wrinkle-free, and traced with a fine pattern of broken blood vessels, the result—he is not shy to admit—of too many hours of work, a bit too much drinking (especially during the hectic days of school integration in Boston), and the overall wear of thirty years as a priest. His age— about the median age of American priests today—and the state of his parish are indicative of the present-day situation (some would call it a crisis) within the Catholic Church.

Faced with a staggering number of churches, buildings, and properties and with an increased number of Catholics nationwide, the church has fewer and increasingly older priests to tend them. In Boston, the number of young men training at St. John's, the archdiocesan seminary, is not nearly enough to replace the men who die, leave, retire, or are incapacitated. There were 1,317 priests in Boston in 1971; as I began to spend time with Father Greer, there were 945. By the year 2000, it is estimated, there will be no more than 400 active priests to serve the archdiocese's 400 parishes. Each year in the archdiocese, an estimated thirty to thirty-five more priests are no longer available for assignment. Although in recent years the seminary has usually managed to produce from twelve to fifteen priests, one year only two were ordained. The seminarians, of course, are the hope, but Father Greer, with his characteristic mixture of frankness and faith, tells any who intern at St. Patrick's, "You have to be nuts to go into the priesthood. It's an awful job. The pay is terrible, the hours are worse. People not only don't look up to you, they look down. You have to love God, and if you don't, it will grind you up. Remember, no trumpets will sound. And you're going to spend more time being a carpenter than a priest."

A modern-day pastor like Father Greer admits that he is at once outmoded and overwhelmed. And, often, confused. As a seminarian, he was trained to give until he literally dropped, and now modern psychology is telling him that this is unhealthy. He was told to keep a tight check on his emotions, and now he is expected to "feel." He looked forward to becoming a pastor and having a role akin to that of a captain aboard ship, but of course Vatican II and the 1960s and 1970s changed all that. In addition, a more vocal and activist pope and an increasingly centralized diocesan bureaucracy have begun to ask more and more of the parishes, inserting the pastor as point man in battles against enemies of moral standards and church law—such as advocates of abortion and birth control and those who would allow non-Catholics and Catholics not in the state of grace to receive Holy Communion. Father Greer finds himself shouldering all the old responsibilities of the pastor, with new ones added, and still has to carry out the time- and energy-consuming rounds and services that occupied him as a young curate.

He is expected to revitalize three quarters of his flock, nominal Catholics who do not attend church regularly; be an inspiring homilist and effective fund-raiser; run an efficient parish; oversee activities from religious education to Alcoholics Anonymous; meet with the many lay committees mandated by Vatican II reforms; let his voice be heard in the community as the key Catholic spokesman; and all the while neglect neither his personal and spiritual growth nor his health. It is a grand juggling act for the priests of Father Greer's generation. And it is to be performed without the power once inherent in the clerical aristocracy, a power that opened doors, closed mouths, and usually paid restaurant and gasoline bills.

For his labors, Father Greer, with thirty years' seniority, makes top scale in the archdiocese, $851 a month. If he worked only a forty-hour week, that would amount to $4.73 an hour. He says as many funeral and wedding Masses, baptizes as many babies, as any of his assistants do. And not only does he no longer preside over meals, frequently he eats alone at the rectory dining room table, or with a retired priest who is in residence at St. Patrick's.

. . .

When Father Greer first drove into Natick in 1985—two and a half years before I met him—to see the parish he had been asked to take, he stopped at the town's main intersection, Central and Main streets, looked up, and instinctively headed toward the dominant and seemingly tallest steeple, covered with perfect, glistening slate shingles and topped with what appeared to be a majestic, gleaming gold cross. To his surprise, he arrived at the Congregational church, and what he had thought was a symbol of Christianity was no more than an elegant weather vane. He was directed farther down Central. Two blocks to the east he came upon a huge billboard advertising bingo every Thursday night, but no sign concerning the church itself. He remembers his initial reaction: "I said, 'Self, something is wrong here.' "

St. Patrick's steeple, octagonally based and finished in tarnished copper, is, in fact, higher than the Congregational church's. (Old parishioners confide that Father McHale, a former pastor, erected the steeple so that the Catholic cross could take its proper place, looking down upon all others.) To Father Greer it looked like a tall, crude, rather narrow dunce's cap. Beneath this embarrassing excess was a huge, sturdy Gothic structure of brick and brownstone with the chapped complexion of an Irish fisherman too long exposed to the North Sea's harshness. Huge, porous openings were visible between the bricks, and cracked, broken, and missing slates formed an incongruous, jagged pattern on the roof. This was St. Patrick's, and it was just as dilapidated inside. In the main church, the paint was dull with age and the carpeting in the aisles was tattered. The tall stained-glass windows had been repaired with no regard for the original colors; there were even obvious misspellings in the memorial inscriptions: "Mijhael" instead of "Michael." In the lower church, where weekday Masses were celebrated, the acoustical tile covering the steam pipes in the ceiling was mottled with rusty stains. The walls seemed alive: the vinyl wall covering undulated in moisture-induced distress.

And to the fastidious Father Greer, whose mother had prophesied during his seminary days, "He may never be the holiest priest, but he'll be the cleanest," the buildings inside and out looked *filthy*.

Administratively, in Father Greer's view, St. Patrick's was in chaos; for years it had not had that staple of church administration, a full-time parish secretary. Fiscally it was a disaster. The average weekly offering was about two dollars per congregant—enough to meet current bills but not enough to finance badly needed repairs, which had been put off for years. People were dunned for a seat offering of twenty-five cents as they arrived for church. Second collections for fuel oil, inflicted almost as a threat with every dip in the temperature from November until spring, evoked little response. Stewardship was practiced in the old-style Catholic way: the yearly financial report, listing names and amounts given, was clearly designed to goad the recalcitrant. Sunday liturgies were lifeless rituals; people hurried out through the vestibule, their heads down, as soon as Mass was over. Though mandated by Vatican II reforms, no homily was delivered at the weekday Masses. Behind his back the pastor was called "The General," both by parishioners and by his priests, who bridled under his authoritarian hand. To him, clergy vacations seemed so much frivolity.

Father Greer had been forewarned. One auxiliary bishop had confided, "Thank God I'm not going there. There are not too many who would want that assignment." St. Patrick's was tired, a parish *in extremis,* and Father Greer sensed that its outward countenance was probably a good reflection of its inner life, despite the assertions of his future parishioners that Natick was the "home of champions." "I had just refurbished another church that was in pretty bad shape, my parish in Hyde Park, and I wasn't looking to do it again," Father Greer told me as we talked about his first impressions of St. Patrick's. "And I couldn't figure out what the personnel boys were thinking about; I'd just been reappointed to my old parish. I was settled in. These days, the ideal parish is simply that: a parish, and a small one at that; no cemetery, school, or hospital to cover. St. Patrick's had them all. These huge parishes used to be sought after, great promotions; today, everybody's trying to duck them. In the old days, the more bricks you had the better. Now everybody wants an igloo. Most pastors want to be senior altar boys."

After seeing St. Patrick's, Father Greer told the clergy personnel director he did not want it.

This is not rare in today's Catholic Church. No longer are priests assigned by fiat, given a week, or days, to conclude all business and duties at one church in order to arrive at the next, as used to be the practice. They are asked. And some senior priests have gone as far as to refuse, consistently, to be named pastor, passing over what was once considered the crowning achievement of diocesan clerical life. "The cardinal's not going to force you, Joe," the personnel director, Father Thomas Oates, said, "but he *needs* you there." As he did with all major decisions in his life, Father Greer sought both temporal advice from fellow priests and spiritual enlightenment through prayer. "I'm not the most loyal son of the church, but we did promise something called obedience, even though it's a little out of fashion these days," he told me. "And I realized the church had been pretty good to me. I was one of the youngest men in the archdiocese to get a pastorate; I once got a four-month sabbatical to go away and study. I felt it was time to give something back. It just seemed to me St. Patrick's was a church that hadn't gotten a fair shake."

Two months later, Father Greer came to St. Patrick's to stay. He smiled benevolently as parishioners told him how fortunate he was to be there in Natick, the town that had given Doug Flutie to football and Joe Coleman to baseball and regularly propelled the high school Red Men to state sports championships. Father Greer responded to their civic pride in his first Sunday homily by telling them he had not wanted to come. "But now that I'm here," he said, "I want it clear that it is not that I won't listen to you—all of you—because I will. But I've come to lead you and not be led by you. That may cause some disagreements now and again." Some of those who attended weekday Masses started grumbling not long after, when the new pastor initiated daily homilies, thus extending a twenty-minute Mass by five minutes. Father Greer relieved his two curates of the almost sacerdotal Sunday morning chore of counting the collection and told them instead to be in the vestibule or on the church steps before and after every Mass. He told them to walk around the parish and, except for their days off, to be available to the people at any time of the day or night. He banished from the church sanctuary to the cellar six majestic but obtrusive candlesticks and a lectern, and moved the other lectern far to the side. This was done in response to liturgical reforms specifying that in the new Mass the altar should be left bare and the readings from Scripture and the intercessory prayers should be done apart from it, so that when the bread and wine were brought forward for the Liturgy of the Eucharist, they would be the focus of attention. Father Greer declared that the parish needed a professional liturgist, an up-to-date religious education program with a paid director, and hundreds of thousands of dollars in repairs to various buildings. He asked each family in the parish to donate about nine dollars a week, the cost of a symbolic loaf of daily bread, which he set at $1.25 ("Just below the price of a good loaf of Jewish rye, which sold for $1.39; after all, these are Catholics"), and promised he would say no more about money.

"And then, there are those larger faith risks in the life of a parish," Father Greer recalled with a wry smile. "Down came the BINGO sign." The Thursday-night games had been bringing in over $60,000 of the church's annual budget of $350,000, but as a weekly reminder that legalized gambling helped to support St. Patrick's, they mortified Father Greer. "I'm certainly not holier than anyone; they could go ahead and play bingo in the school basement—but a sign proclaiming it on my front lawn!"

Bingo enthusiasts were outraged, but in a few weeks, a parishioner pledged the cost of a ST. PATRICK'S sign for the front of the church, and Father Greer felt his leap of faith had been justified. He was on his way. As he saw it, "Natick is basically a conservative area, but we have great diversity in the parish: the old "townies" and the swinging liberals, senior citizens and the high-tech crowd out on Route 128, the Blue Army bunch who think Vatican II is heresy and see the Virgin Mary popping up all over the world, twenty-five-year-old kids who wear scapulars and pro-lifers ready to excommunicate everybody. Some welcomed the changes I brought, and for others I was taking away their Linus blanket. I see the kernel of the diocese as the parish, and the family as the kernel of the parish. I wanted to hold up and buttress the family and all the old values that seem to be ground under today, and at the same time try to bring people into the cadence of the modern church. The pastor's life is a public life, and if you can't stand the heat, you shouldn't be doing it. You've got to take the pokes with the strokes. And anyhow, what could be worse than everybody agreeing with you?"

The changes came almost weekly. No longer did priests harangue the faithful from the pulpit for the second collections for which the

Catholic Church is legendary. Instead, a low-key note in the bulletin explained the need for funds. The meaning of the sign of peace—the moment of offering symbolic friendship and forgiveness to fellow worshipers—was explained, and while some parishioners continued to stand stiffly in place, more began to turn to their neighbors, offering a smile, a nod, or a handshake. Father Greer often eased the introduction of his innovations with personal stories, often self-deprecating. "My father never knew the Mass prayers; he just said a rosary. So much for the Greer family's liturgical input. But the church is changing; it's a good thing not only to worship together and know the prayers but to acknowledge that fellow over there in the corner."

He planned a half-dozen socials during the year, fund-raisers to be sure, but nicely packaged ones—enjoyable nights out. He talked about projecting the parish's needs rather than waiting to react when a crisis struck. A new roof went up on the church, a new boiler arrived in the basement. His priests were seen walking about the parish. Committees for liturgy and education and finance were formed. Some parishioners greeted Father Greer with a smile and a pat on the back after Sunday Mass; others wrote to Bernard Cardinal Law, the archbishop, protesting the destructive clerical tornado that had been visited upon Natick.

About a year and a half into his pastorship at St. Patrick's, just as the physical work on parish structures was getting under way and a new spirit seemed to be enkindling the people, Father Greer's illness was diagnosed. Parishioners wondered what effect this ominous disease would have on him, but once he was released from the hospital and had started his chemotherapy, Father Greer resumed the pace they had begun to expect of him.

Father Greer was appointed, as pastors are today in Boston, for a six-year period. That was the interval the parishioners generally thought he had in mind for the overhaul of their church. But once he was diagnosed with multiple myeloma, Father Greer sensed he had a different timetable to meet.

2

Mine is a parish like all the rest. They're all alike. Those of today I mean. I was saying so only yesterday . . . that good and evil are probably evenly distributed, but on such a low plain, very low indeed! Or if you like they lie one over the other; like oil and water they never mix.

To see what a pastor like Father Greer does, there is no need to choose a special day—or night—in which his work will appear more complex or dramatic than usual. A Tuesday morning in August, traditionally a slow month in parish life, will do for a start. August is a month when pastors perform routine functions but are usually assured ample time for rest, reading, and plenty of golf before the onset of the busy fall schedule; a sort of modified vacation.

It is 8:40 A.M. and the windows are open to warm, moist morning air in the third-floor common room at St. Patrick's rectory. This is a sunny, comfortable place whose furniture, rugs, wallpaper, and draperies are done in the muted rusts and browns which practical bachelors might be expected to choose. On the table between two Berkline Wallaway reclining chairs are a telephone and a remote-control activator for the twenty-one-inch television set that sits across the room. Three men are present for morning prayer: Father Greer; one of his two assistants, Father Neil Mullaney, age forty-three (the other, Father Joseph Rossi, age twenty-nine, is on vacation); and Monsignor Joseph Mahoney, age seventy-nine, the former pastor of St. Patrick's, now retired but in residence at the parish (a practice that has since been discontinued in the Boston archdiocese because of conflicts that have arisen between former and present men in charge).

The wind is blowing from the northwest this morning, bringing with it both the pleasant yeasty aroma from the huge Wonder Bread factory down near Route 9 and another layer of the fine dust that drives the housekeeper to despair. Just below the windows a crane is at work, dropping its jaw some thirty feet to crush mounds of bricks, lath, and framing that a few days earlier it had toppled with a wrecking ball. Natick firemen had been present during the demolition, but today there are no streams of water to keep the dust from flying wherever the winds of Natick may blow it.

Father Greer looks out over what until recently had been a block consisting primarily of commercial buildings. These businesses— the Natick Pizza Palace, the Dog and Groom Shop, a drugstore, a doughnut shop, and the Colonial movie theater—had been eclipsed by shopping centers, and downtown Natick customers had no longer supported them. Father Greer's features have that amazing elasticity I noted in our first meeting: the face, so vigorous and expectant when he greeted his priests this morning, has now turned gloomy and distant as he stands by the window. "I understand the scrap metal will be shipped to Europe," he states flatly. He returns to his chair and opens his breviary to a place marked by a red ribbon.

Father Greer has been up since shortly before six. Part of his night's sleep was sacrificed for an emergency call at Leonard Morse Hospital to administer the last rites to a victim of a motorcycle accident, a nineteen-year-old boy who died before the priest arrived. Since rising, Father Greer has spent a half hour meditating on the Scripture passage that will form the basis of his Sunday homily; has read a page or two of Dom Marmion's *Christ, The Ideal of the Priest* (a book from his seminary days, now decidedly out of vogue because of its narrow focus on the private spirituality of the priest); has showered, shaved, and opened the mail he didn't get to yesterday. He is particularly tired this morning; the previous day was more grueling than most: he drove into Boston to battle the Metropolitan Boston Transit Authority over the church parking lot their commuters are using, which the MBTA refuses to help maintain; spent time with a reformed drug addict who had lapsed; juggled Mass, hospital, and duty-day schedules so that he and his reduced staff could cover both St. Patrick's and a neighboring parish, priestless for the next few days because of vacations; tackled a major physical plant problem (oil tanks behind the church may be leaking) and a thorny administrative one (the contract for his parish bulletin seems to unduly favor the printer); and made sick calls at Leonard Morse Hospital, which were extended for an hour because of a panicky woman who kept screaming, "I don't want to die" as he tried to administer the Sacrament of the Sick.

This morning Father Greer has taken his chemotherapy medication, capsules of Alkeran and prednisone—which did not nauseate him, as they sometimes did—and has had a large bowl of bran cereal and a cup of coffee for breakfast.

> My song is of mercy and justice;
> I sing to you, O Lord.
> I will walk in the way of perfection.
> Oh when, Lord, will you come?
> I will walk with blameless heart within my house;
> I will not set before my eyes whatever is base.

The powerful and reassuring words of Psalm 101 are read alternately by the three men, whose voices compete with the diesel engine on the crane as it strains to hoist the larger pieces of twisted I beams it has dislodged. The phone rings; during these fifteen minutes at St. Patrick's it goes unanswered. Soon after he came to the parish, Father Greer told his fellow priests he wanted to begin the day with prayers said in common. ("Despite our weaknesses and regardless of any personal tensions or animosities, it unifies us as priests and specifies what we do," he explained to me later. "It's a time to forgive each other. We are a small community within a larger community, and we need to ask the Lord's blessing for the day. Often it's the only time we get together; it's a chance to catch up on what each of us is doing.") This practice seems a small move toward building that sense of community, but as Father Mullaney told me, "If St. Patrick's isn't the only parish in Boston where it's done, it's one of the few."

Once the prayers are over, Father Greer does not use this morning gathering, as might be expected of an efficient manager, for "morning reports." Father Greer gives his priests wide leeway in how they employ themselves; he jokingly calls it a "fearful liberty." Rather, the time after morning office provides an opportunity for brief comments on such random items as the fortunes of whatever Boston sports team is in season, Father Mullaney's charismatic conference, Father Rossi's well-attended trip with parish youth, Monsignor Mahoney's vacation plans. This morning Father Greer mentions the phone call he received the night before from an elderly Jesuit who, in asking permission for a graveside interment at the parish cemetery, made it clear he didn't want to do it himself. "I could hear it in the funeral director's voice too, so I said I'd go over," Father Greer says. " 'Father I'll-Do-Also' steps in again. A day-old baby. I just hope it wasn't the first child." He shakes his head. "Not even our parishioners."

Father Greer is not unduly irritated by the funeral director's request. He knows his institution all too well and how work can be avoided on grounds of protocol, and also that people can be alienated or frightened away from their church at vulnerable times such as these. Rather than ask the questions that could easily release him from such tasks, he usually says yes. He claims it's just easier that way.

At a few minutes before nine, Father Greer is in the sacristy, robed in a white polyester alb tied at the waist with a cincture, a green stole draped over his neck. He takes a last look at the Scripture readings for the day and recites the five petitions headed "Most Profitable to Recite Before and After Communion" from a well-thumbed copy of *Priestly Prayers for the Holy Hour*, another no-longer-popular devotional text. Such moments of reflection before a service are somewhat new; in his early days in the priesthood the commonly accepted practice was "sheet to alb": only minutes divided time in bed from time at the altar. There was no need for preparation; the Mass was in Latin and uniform, and a homily was considered unnecessary.

He walks alone out to the altar and turns to greet the thirty or forty people, most of them elderly, who are scattered about the lower church, which seats six hundred. A fluorescent light, giving its last, flickers over a statue of St. Patrick to the left of the altar.

A man has begun to mutter his prayers audibly, which he will continue to do throughout the Mass. Father Greer looks out over his faithful, who are standing in straight-backed pews seemingly constructed to ensure maximum discomfort whether the congregation is standing or sitting, with kneelers whose wafer-thin pads offer only a hint of relief. Among the worshipers this morning—and he knows each face—are those who have written to the archbishop asking that Father Greer be immediately replaced, as well as those who think he is the best thing to happen to St. Patrick's in decades.

Father Greer says Mass in a reverent yet relaxed manner, his tone at all but the most holy of moments little different from the timbre and pitch of his normal speaking voice. The overall impression is of a man talking to the worshipers more than of one presiding over them. He does not rush the prayers, respecting all the moments set aside for silence. He spurns the classic shortcuts of combining the offertory prayers for the bread and wine instead of pronouncing them separately and eliminating the Prayer of the Faithful. These are small but well-known economies utilized by some priests to whittle a few minutes from the Liturgy and please those worshipers who, while they want to attend Mass daily, are happy to see it offered as expeditiously as possible. Father Greer officiates with priestly dignity, not the efficiency of a clerical short-order cook.

His homily this morning is based on a well-known but widely misunderstood scriptural passage from St. Matthew, "It is easier for a camel to pass through the eye of a needle than for a rich man to enter the kingdom of heaven." In four minutes, the priest offers a short lesson in Bible interpretation, adding a dollop of history. The "needle's eye," he tells the tiny congregation, was, at the time of Christ, a low gate or small opening in a city wall. It was the last entrance to be closed at night, and for reasons of security it was large enough for only a single person to get through.

And then a message to take with them: "Narrow? Difficult? Of course it's difficult. Look up at that cross. That wasn't easy either, my friends. But here was a love so great that nothing short of giving His life for us would do." There is no burning sincerity in his voice even as he reaches the point in his homily that many a preacher would weight with emotion. "And what is our narrow gate? Illness?

Scorn?" He smiles broadly. "Parish life? We all carry a cross, but we all have Him inside us. That is a strength and a love equal to any hardship, isn't it? 'Father, forgive them, for they know not what they do.' We live with each other's sinfulness. Be loving. Don't beat yourself up. Don't beat the next guy up."

There is no demand for immediate conversion; a conversational tone has prevailed throughout, one that might be used over a dinner table to make a point.

Back at the rectory after a trip to the bank to deposit two sacks containing Sunday's collection—the trustee who usually does this is on vacation—Father Greer slides behind the desk in his office, a corner room on the second floor, looks at the first of a small stack of notes, and returns a phone call from the previous day. The Delphi Academy in Cambridge has outgrown its quarters and may be interested in renting part of St. Patrick's grade school. He asks if the academy has any religious affiliation and the caller says it does not. Yes, he understands they are pressed for time, and he squeezes a note about the appointment, in tiny print, onto his desktop calendar following one at two-thirty, "Talk to neighbors about clubhouse," and preceding one at four, "Spiritual Director."

"Delphi? Delphi? Doesn't ring a bell." Not a man to go into any meeting unprepared, Father Greer reaches for the archdiocesan directory. "Let's see what Geno has to say about these Delphi folks." He puts in a call to Father Eugene Sullivan, the superintendent of Boston's parochial schools. "When did he resign?" Father Greer greets the news with a weary nod. "And what is *sister's* name, the new superintendent?"

The church secretary, Janet Hamilton, brings in a five-inch pile of morning mail, half of which Father Greer disposes directly into the wastebasket without opening the envelopes—the Paulist Press, a mission in Africa, an office supply house, a computer software company are among those whose offers or pleas will not be heard. He separates the other mail into stacks: one will go to the church office—items such as donations and requests for baptismal certificates; another he will read later; a third is invoices. "A good morning," he says. "Got through with only eighteen hundred bucks in bills."

By the time Janet buzzes to tell him "The oil tank man is here,"

Father Greer has made four calls to various chancery officials and priest friends, none of whom have any information about the Delphi Academy, and has quickly scanned *Catholic Quotes*, a monthly magazine of devotional and liturgical material, for a Marian quote for this week's church bulletin. He tears out a page to take downstairs with him.

Richard Horan, the president and part owner of Hughes Oil Company, and Father Greer were classmates at Boston College High School and Boston College, and the two men shake hands warmly. "The oil tanks for the church and school might not be leaking at all, might be just fine, but they don't pass the new pressure test Natick wants," Horan explains. "But don't feel bad; the test is impossible to perform accurately. This is the environmental age. It costs."

"Okay, Dickie, what are we looking at?"

"We're looking at a twenty-five-thousand-dollar job to dig up the old tanks, dispose of them—that costs, too—and replace them with state-of-the-art Sti-P3 tanks." Father Greer grins warily. "When Natick comes back to test it in five years, will they still be state of the art?" he asks. Horan produces a convincing color brochure on the Sti-P3 tank and Father Greer tells him he won't be able to pay for a few months, until a certificate of deposit comes due. "But can you get moving on the tanks as soon as possible?" the priest says. "I'm hoping to convince our beloved MBTA to pave the parking lot over one of the tanks and we don't want to ask those generous souls twice. Commuters have been using that lot for twenty-five years, and it's about time a few pennies came our way to help maintain it."

It is typical of Father Greer to do business with a man like Horan, who is a classmate, Irish, and a Catholic. For a man like Father Greer, who has lived here all his life, Boston is, after all, a small town, half of whose residents are Catholic and the majority of those Irish. During nearly thirty years of ordained life, Father Greer has seen school friends, parishioners, and ex-priests go into most of the businesses a pastor must call on, and he usually prefers to deal with a person he knows rather than one who might come in with the lowest price or the fanciest sales presentation. And he is not reluctant to go back to them wearing his Judas shirt to extract gift certificates, merchandise, or sports tickets for his raffles.

After seeing Horan out, Father Greer walks into the kitchen to tell Anna Caruso, the early-shift cook, that he's ready for lunch. But by the time the fruit salad with a scoop of raspberry sherbet is served, he has been interrupted three times: a chancery official calls to say he has not been able to find out anything about the Delphi Academy; a wealthy Boston College classmate says he's good for his usual two tickets to a Patriots game; and William Gately, a Natick funeral director, provides details of the baby's interment. While he has Gately on the line, Father Greer quotes him the new annual fee for the funeral home's listing in the weekly parish bulletin: "Two thousand bucks; is that okay, Billy? Knocking it down from twenty-four hundred this year. New printer; got to watch this guy, but you're getting a bargain." The sherbet sags into the fruit salad.

As Father Greer makes his way toward the dining room, Paul Fitzgerald, the St. Patrick's cemetery foreman, tells him that the hunks of sidewalk and the boulders hastily used as landfill years ago in an unused section now have to be excavated as the backhoe can't move them to dig graves. He also asks if the pastor has decided what to do with the Sacred Heart statue. "No hands on it, wires sticking out," Father Greer replies. "Saw it yesterday. I said, 'You're in pretty tough shape, kid; not even worth sending you to the manicurist.' Maybe we should leave them off, like that statue in Germany after the war: 'Lend me your hands.' I want to get a St. Patrick, so I'll give you the Sacred Heart from the front of the church—every church in Natick has a Sacred Heart in front; must have been on sale. Let's wait for the uproar from the faithful when I move *their* statue."

Father Greer finally bolts his lunch just before Christina Wilhelm walks by the dining room, ready for her one o'clock appointment.

Father Greer is, as he puts it, "murdered" by the number of meetings he has to attend with church groups. Many of them, he feels, could be handled with a phone call, and he tries to limit them as best he can. Although in the spirit of Vatican II he does rely on the advice and consent of his parishioners and gives them great latitude in the various committees, he has not fostered a parish council, supposedly the cornerstone of the new church partnership between clergy and laity. He simply found the parish council system inefficient in dealing with day-to-day church problems and a waste of time. "Talkers, not doers, that's what it was" is his assessment.

"And quite frankly, as I looked at who was talking and who was doing, I had another thought: this church would have gotten a lot further if Christ had chosen twelve *women* as his Apostles."

Mrs. Wilhelm represents a new trend in the Catholic Church—the professional liturgist—as well as a ten-thousand-dollar annual expenditure for St. Patrick's, which is among the approximately 5 percent of churches employing such a person. She is an energetic woman in her early fifties, a classical pianist and accomplished accompanist. In the pre–Vatican II church there was little room for a person with her talents; the Mass was unvarying throughout the world—a point of pride with Catholics—and an organist who was also the choir director chose the hymns for each service from a limited and approved group. The worshipers in the pews were passive participants. But now, although the form of the Mass is set, there are many options open to Mrs. Wilhelm. She selects music appropriate to the various feast days or to tie in with the Scripture readings, by composers ranging from Bach, Mozart, and César Franck to contemporary composers. She may use an adult choir, a children's choir, or an instrumental group in addition to the cantor, who leads the congregation in song. She works with Father Greer on whatever is needed to make St. Patrick's services more conducive to worship. And she also has charge of the lectors—the laypeople who read the Scripture selections and lead the intercessory prayers—the altar boys, and the extraordinary ministers who help the priest distribute Holy Communion. In short, she oversees everyone who has a role in the Liturgy except the priest. All of these jobs either did not exist before Vatican II or were handled by the ample number of nuns, brothers, and priests.

This afternoon's talk begins not with Brahms or Bach but with the ushers. "They hang around the holy water font like they were at a bar having a beer with the boys," says Father Greer. "People are walking into church, maybe had a fight at home, and if somebody just said hello, it might get them over the hump." Mrs. Wilhelm agrees and will speak to the ushers. She moves on to the first item on her list: a desire to revamp the upper church sanctuary so that she could bring her choir down from their elegant loft into the midst of the people. "I just think people will respond better—sing more—if the choir is visible to them," she says. Father Greer nods.

"We've got the audio, now we got to work on the visual. Let's go over to the church and see what we can do. But we've got to do it quick; I've got stuff backing up."

St. Patrick's upper church, a soaring paean to the Early English Gothic architecture of the thirteenth century and the pride of Natick when it was dedicated in 1902, is an extremely unsuitable setting for the Liturgy introduced by Vatican II. There is an elegant carved Carrara marble altar rail which, before Vatican II, demarcated the holy area where the mysteries were performed in Latin by a priest with his back to the congregation. Its presence now is an affront to the sense of community the council sought to foster. Side altars to the Virgin Mary and St. Joseph are no longer used. Twenty-five years ago, the main altar was repositioned away from the back wall of the church, so that the priest could say Mass facing the congregation, but it was not moved far enough forward to allow ease of movement. Worse, the tabernacle, containing consecrated Hosts, is on a shelf on the wall behind the altar, so that Father Greer must necessarily turn his back on the Christ he is there to honor and invoke. Father Greer, who was on the archdiocesan liturgical commission and understands modern worship, is well aware of the problems; Mrs. Wilhelm, who has just returned from a Liturgy workshop in Washington burning with zeal, is appalled anew by the setup, which she has deplored since she was hired a year ago.

They stand in the chancel and quickly agree on the removal of a section of the communion rail. About marble, Father Greer is open-minded; he balks at electricity. "I know you need outlets for the mike and all that stuff, but let's see how this goes before we go further. I just got hit with a twenty-five-thousand-dollar whopper this morning." Mrs. Wilhelm eyes the chancel. "I guess we can do it with extension cords for a while," she says. Father Greer glances at his watch. "Just don't make it look like a summer stock company with cords all over the floor." Mrs. Wilhelm smiles. "A piano?" He feigns exasperation. "No more stuff up here, or else it'll look like a drawing room in the Museum of Fine Arts and not an altar. Okay, okay, see if it fits. Now let me get out of here so I can go out into the neighborhood and let them chew me up when I tell them what we're up to with the clubhouse."

While Jim Cuddy, the director of the South Middlesex Opportunity Council, waits in the rectory parlor, Father Greer goes into the small office across the hall, closes the door, and hears the confession of a woman who had been waiting for him. Another woman, the one who had complained over the phone of being "environmentally poisoned" by her landlord, appears with her daughter, whom she claims has suffered from uncontrolled hemorrhaging, and she has a sheaf of documentation. Father Greer listens for a few minutes and, pointing to Cuddy and explaining their mission, asks her to return the next day. As she is leaving, he asks if she has a place to stay that night. She does. He presses a folded twenty-dollar bill into her hand.

Then he and Cuddy walk out the back door of the rectory into the wilting heat of a humid summer afternoon. The back of Father Greer's black clerical shirt, which has been alternately soaked and allowed to dry, depending on the location of his work thus far today—his office is air-conditioned—shows a roughly circular white perspiration stain. By the time he reaches the first home, on the edge of the church parking lot and next door to the clubhouse, the shirt is already damp, the whiteness once again invisible.

On the porch, Father Greer turns to Cuddy, a handsome man in his early forties. "Ready to be fed to the lions, Jim?" Cuddy has devised a plan to remake St. Patrick's decrepit, condemned clubhouse—which was once a meeting place for now-defunct men's and women's groups such as the Holy Name Society and the Sodality but more recently has become a haven for the local pigeon population—into a halfway house for homeless people, most of whom have received counseling and treatment for drug and alcohol dependency at a shelter in nearby Framingham. Father Greer had once considered tearing down the structure because of its many building code violations but had found that, because it was so close to the sidewalk, it could not, under current zoning laws, have been replaced. St. Patrick's no longer has use for such a building—nor does Father Greer need another "program" in residence. He already houses, within the rectory or the school, everything from craft workshops to Overeaters Anonymous, in addition to various church groups. And although Cuddy will hire a full-time resident manager, there is no program at St. Patrick's that does not eventually require a pastor's time. Still, the proposal offers a practical solution for two long-standing problems: the house will be renovated at no cost to the church, and Natick will have a place for ten of the working poor who would not otherwise be able to live in the community. Father Greer's involvement might perhaps be written off as pure pragmatism, but as Jim Cuddy had found, not one of the dozens of other Catholic churches within his area was willing to exercise such pragmatism with respect to any of its properties. While the parishes of the Archdiocese of Boston are rich in buildings, many unused or underutilized these days, there are few priests willing to wend their way through the tortuous bureaucracies of Church and State to carry out such projects. They are time-consuming, and there are attendant legal problems, as well as the risk of failure and embarrassment. Priests feel they are already overworked.

Affordable housing is one of Father Greer's great crusades, although it is not one in which he has been particularly successful. The demolition going on beneath the third-floor window where he gathered with his priests to pray this morning is a perfect example of one of his failures. Andrew Lane (always referred to by Father Greer in conversation as *Mr.* Andrew Lane) assembled most of the properties, including a few single-family homes, within the block bounded by East Central, Hayes, and Clarendon streets and South Avenue, and laid before the Natick town council his plan to demolish much of the block to make room for a 160-unit condominium. Father Greer heatedly voiced his disapproval at a planning board meeting after he found that the smallest units would sell for $180,000. He noted that of the last twenty parish couples he had married, only two had been able to afford housing in Natick, and neither of them would have had the means to buy a unit in Mr. Lane's proposed Natick Park. Father Greer joined other voices to protest that while Natick was rapidly becoming a boon to developers and a bedroom community for the ever-growing number of DINKs, less financially able citizens—the elderly and especially families with children, Natick's backbone—were being neglected.

When the plan was approved, as he had expected it would be, Father Greer took the next step. He paid a call on Mr. Andrew Lane, a Natick native who was raised a Catholic, and asked him to set aside some units at lower cost for senior citizens or others of limited means and to keep them in a trust so that their market value

would not be driven up and they would remain affordable housing.
Mr. Lane was cordial to Father Greer, but he flatly refused his
request, saying it was economically impossible. He offered instead,
as best Father Greer can recall his words, to " 'come up to the
church and see if I can help you with something.' " To Father
Greer it was an insult, a pat on the head, an offer to buy some
needed equipment, make a donation, whatever Father wanted, to
ensure peace. It may not have been a bribe, but it certainly was not
what Father Greer was after, and he told Mr. Lane that that would
not be necessary. "And this was the man who a year before wanted
to buy my school and turn it into more condos—or a parking lot!"
On that occasion Father Greer had said, "Mr. Lane, what do you
think you see? A piece of hay sticking out from between my teeth?"

The porch door opens and Father Greer and Cuddy are led into
Mrs. Katherine Argir's spotlessly clean kitchen. She is an elderly
widow and not a parishioner. After a comment on the hot weather—
"Even the nuns aren't happy on a day like this"—Father Greer
presents his case. "We preach a lot about giving shelter to the
homeless, but we don't do too much in Natick, this supposed 'home
of champions.' Seems like half-million-dollar estates and those fancy
condos are winning out. So we're trying to do this little bit. These
are our people, from Natick, maybe Framingham, this area, and
they've fallen on some tough times, lost a home, maybe were drinking too much or taking drugs. But they're straightened out and
they'll be living in the house for up to two years while they go to
school or participate in job training. No drinking allowed. No retarded folks, either."

"Father," Mrs. Argir interrupts.

Father Greer is ready for her rejoinder.

"The retarded are people too, Father."

The priest and Cuddy exchange a grin. There are three other
calls to make and they go similarly well; the clubhouse's new use
gets a far better response than the priest had expected. The roofing
contractor and dentist have no problems with it, and the last woman,
a parishioner whom Father Greer knows is not one of his backers,
actually terms it "a good idea. It gets kind of lonesome around here
at night. It'll be good to see more people."

The two men walk back toward the rectory, not basking in their success but immediately moving on to the details of archdiocesan approvals, the merits of various general contractors, and Cuddy's fund-raising plans to pay for the renovation. "They always amaze me," Father Greer suddenly interjects.

"Who?" Cuddy asks.

"People. A basic goodness out there, Jim."

Perhaps—Father Greer would surely scoff at the idea—there was something else at work. As he talks, it is not difficult to believe him, feel his rectitude, and want to cooperate with him. A compelling quality emanates from him, the consequence of a simple trait: Father Greer is not a man who appears to be saying any more or less than what he is.

The representatives of the Delphi Academy—three unsmiling woman similarly attired in faded, overlarge housedresses—arrive half an hour late. They tour the school building and Father Greer tells them in some detail about the school's closing. "The nuns got tired of teaching and wanted to work in what we used to call relevant ministries," he says. "Off they went to the inner city and their apartments, and most of them kept on going, right out of religious life. I went for dinner one night to one of their apartments and asked for a Manhattan and got it served in a frappé glass. One of the sisters had this bandage on her head. She'd toasted herself with a curling iron. Poor darlings; they were so naïve."

Father Greer is smiling, but his audience sees no humor in his tale.

"So anyhow, in 1974 St. Patrick's dumped seven hundred kids on the Natick public school system overnight and closed the doors. Used to be the backbone of the parish. Sad. We use it a couple of afternoons a week for our CCD, Confraternity of Christian Doctrine; you know, religious education. One night for bingo. Otherwise here it is, empty." After the tour, Father Greer still knows no more about their school than what he was told initially over the phone: that Delphi is a private, nonreligious institution with an emphasis on ethical behavior. He has received what he feels are evasive answers to his questions about the school's underpinnings, and his lack of enthusiasm about renting to the women is becoming apparent.

The women do not call back, and it is just as well. In a few days he will find out that Delphi's curriculum is influenced by the

Church of Scientology—not an organization within Father Greer's pantheon of acceptable belief systems.

By four he is headed, late, for his monthly half-hour appointment with his spiritual director, Father Joseph Payne, a Dominican priest and the prior at St. Stephen's Priory in Dover. It is to him that Father Greer goes to confess and to discuss the state of his soul, and it is Father Payne's task not only to direct him in paths of holiness but also, now that the church has a better appreciation of its clergy's needs, to address his psychological and physical well-being as well.

Father Greer returns shortly after five and goes upstairs to his living quarters—a comfortable three-room suite on the second floor of the rectory consisting of his office, a living room, and a bedroom. During his customary cocktail hour, he serves Manhattans made with good sweet vermouth and a serviceable, inexpensive bourbon. With shoes off and collar loosened, he tells of the session. "Father Payne asked how much time I spent in quiet reflection today and I had to admit it was—pathetically—only minutes. He asked if I thought that was enough, and, well, I didn't have to answer. When confronted, I have to admit I'm not praying enough. The good Lord got another punch in the trunks today. He asked what I thought God was saying with the myeloma, and I told him it's the same thing I tell sick people: give in; let go; slow down. Listen to God.

"But it's hard; I feel better than I have in such a long time. That chemo has really put me together. And I'm like a racehorse. After all, this is what I was trained to do. There's so much to be done before . . . well, just before."

3

A true priest is never loved, get that through your head.

It is nightfall a few days later, and the traffic that jams East Central Street in front of St. Patrick's during the workday slows to a trickle. The low roar of engines is gone and the theme from *Finlandia* resounds dully and slightly off key from the carillon within the church's steeple. Natick is once again the unexceptional, quiet suburban town it was before high technology and Boston's thriving economy transformed it into a desirable—and expensive—place to live. The streetlights along East Central illuminate only the lower half of the church and even less of the school, set back as it is from the sidewalk, but the white-shingled parish house, its blemishes and rust stains forgiven, glimmers in the harsh glow—a beacon, a presence, like a spiritual fire station whose occupants are ready to respond to all calls, all needs. At least for now.

Father Greer is on duty—something former pastors of St. Patrick's did not have to endure—and has appointments with two couples.

Evening appointments at the rectory, a long-standing tradition, have become more prevalent as more women have gone into the work force and fewer people can come to see their priests during the day. It is not that Father Greer works every evening—he does not. He is frequently out to dinner with fellow priests or visiting friends from former parishes, like the Hajjars in Braintree (Linda Hajjar affectionately calls him "Jo-Jo"). Or he may be off to Dom the barber's house in Mattapan for his biweekly haircut, which Dom does for free. Or he might have an evening social event or a dinner engagement, perhaps at a Boston restaurant, with some active St. Patrick's parishioners like the Garveys or the Barrys. He is not much of a moviegoer, nor does he enjoy plays, ballet, opera, or other cultural events. A Celtics or Red Sox game is more to his liking, but he is offered more tickets than he uses and gives most of them away.

As he waits in his second-floor living room to be summoned downstairs for the first appointment, Father Greer is on the phone. In the background Tom Brokaw presents the seven o'clock news. The book Father Greer had hoped to read tonight, Rembert Weakland's *All God's People: Catholic Identity After the Vatican Council*, lies open to a page early in the first chapter.

The woman who claimed her landlord's heating system had poisoned her daughter and herself, making it necessary for them to move out, not only is homeless but has an apartment full of furniture that may end up on the street any day. Father Greer has already provided her with a few nights' lodging at a local shelter, as well as food vouchers and some cash, but the furniture is not as easy a problem to solve. He is calling a friend, a former parishioner, in the moving and storage business. "Wouldn't be for too long," Father Greer says. "Oh, you're jammed to the rafters? Okay, let me see where else we can put the poor dear's things."

It has not been the worst of days up to this point, in Father Greer's assessment, but hardly the best. The words "shit" and "fuck" were found scrawled on the back of a pew, and a deposit of human feces was left in the monsignor's confessional. Since the rug was stolen two months earlier and the St. Vincent de Paul poor box was broken into last month, Father Greer has been battling within himself as to whether or not to close the church during the day—St. Patrick's is the only Natick church still open all day for those who wish to pray. A parishioner had stopped Father Greer after Mass and demanded he stop allowing funerals at "her" nine o'clock Mass; this "violated" her experience of Liturgy. Another member of the congregation had paid for a fellow parishioner's trip to Fatima for a cure, thought she might have been bilked, and wanted Father Greer to investigate. A good portion of his afternoon was spent with a man recently released from the state penitentiary at Billerica who needed food, money, and a job. A huge man with arm muscles that stretched the elastic of his knit shirt, he offered a limp excuse when Father Greer said there was immediate work available as a grave-digger in St. Patrick's cemetery.

But there were better moments. A woman with extensive religious education experience agreed to be his new CCD director, and Dr. Desforges called to say that his blood counts were steadily improving and he could soon discontinue his chemotherapy. He was able to get in a half-mile swim at the Natick YMCA. No bills came in the mail.

The buzzer on his phone sounds. The first appointment is here. Tom Brokaw is signing off.

Father Greer greets a man and woman in their early twenties and ushers them into the small office across from the first-floor parlor. Although he is slightly built, the young man has the oversized hands and thick, dirt-rimmed fingers of a mechanic. His lank blond hair is freshly washed but errantly combed and trails over his collar. He has come here to acknowledge his failure in an earlier marriage, in the hope of obtaining an annulment. He wants, with the church's approval, to marry the young woman who sits so nervously beside him, grasping his hand as he begins his tale of young passion and eventual sordidness.

"My wife and I were from different backgrounds, Father," the young man says. "I was working-class and she came from better. I was working in a gas station and she'd ride down to get air for her bicycle. She was cutting classes; she dropped out. She went to hairdresser school but she never could hold a job. We messed around and so she was pregnant. We had to get married, so we did. The baby came and we needed to save money and she wanted to party. She just walked out and left me with the baby. Then one day she picked him up at day care and brought him back to where she was living with this guy. There were a lot of guys; I could make a list."

A picture of Cardinal Law gazes majestically over Father Greer's shoulder and down onto the young man and his fiancée, a slender girl with frizzy brunet hair, dressed with schoolgirl simplicity in starched white blouse and dark skirt. Father Greer looks over their annulment application, pencils a few notes onto a pad, and looks up. His eyes are sad, knowing. Perhaps there is a trace of disap-

pointment in them, even some anger. He is a firm believer in the
sanctity and indissolubility of marriage. He often preaches about it
at St. Patrick's. And he is an ardent advocate of the nuclear family,
refusing to make his school into a day care center, although such
centers at other parishes are proven money-makers and perhaps
magnets for young couples, who then attend church. He believes
day care centers are one of the more obvious shortcomings of contemporary life (which he groups under his "law of substitution")
because they substitute paid care for parental care, tearing further
at the fabric of the family.

The room is deathly still.

"You thought with your body and not with your mind or soul,
young man," Father Greer says quietly. "Now there's a child. And
a dead marriage. Not a proud legacy, is it?"

The young woman kicks her intended husband's shin, out of
Father Greer's view.

The young man caps his hands over his knees, slouches forward,
and looks down. Father Greer turns to the young woman, and she,
too, peers dejectedly at the floor. Once eye contact is lost owing to
his opening volley, the priest's face seems to clear, taking on a kind
of benign neutrality. "But you did. That's over. You're looking at
your ecclesiastical lawyer, for better or worse. Let's see what we can
do about the rest of your lives."

After a series of questions and a careful editing of their application,
making subjects and predicates agree and fractured words become
whole, Father Greer reads them his longhand covering letter, which
will accompany the application. It is a concise and simply stated
story of two careless children marrying in order to legitimize an
impending birth; its key and canonically decisive point is that in
reality there was no marriage because they were incapable of handling themselves in life situations and were therefore unable to
contract a marriage.

"These annulment petitions are going in like gangbusters, so I
don't know how long it will take. Rome doesn't like a diocese
breaking any records for volume. It's going to cost two or three
hundred bucks, none of which goes to Father Greer; I'll be sending
it right along to the marriage tribunal. Say a prayer that when those
priests in the tribunal receive this, a breeze will blow in on their

thick skulls that will convince them God's mercy is greater than the rules men have made. Now let's see how many stamps this rocket needs to get it in the air," he says, leaving the room. He returns, after weighing the letter in the church office, with the appropriate number of stamps. "Realize they may turn it down," he tells them, ushering the couple to the front door.

"But I've never had one come back."

In the darkness of the vestibule, the streetlight, shining through the four tiny windows over the front door, illuminates their faces; their expressions have been transposed from worried frowns to tentative smiles by Father Greer's parting sentence.

The second couple, a bit older than the first and obviously better off, are more casually dressed: she in culottes, he in beige cotton shorts and a laundry-starched white oxford cloth shirt open to mid-chest. They are positively beaming.

Father Greer poses the first question he asks every couple about to be married:

"How much do you folks make?

"Sorry to be so blunt, but I find—and you don't need to be a genius to come up with this—that money is a weak sister to faith and the cause of more marriages going on the rocks. I guess what I'm saying is, Can you afford to get married?"

Their prenuptial glow is undimmed by such brashness. He makes fifty-five thousand dollars in high-tech sales, and she forty-five thousand dollars in pharmaceutical sales. From here on, in Father Greer's quick way of encapsulating people, he will remember them as "the hundred-thousand-dollar couple."

Their responses to the priest's further questions, as he fills out the two-sided archdiocesan marriage form, make up a story quite different from that of the previous couple. These are children of the mobile middle class, who have moved so frequently that they have difficulty remembering all their former addresses. It is the new generation of Catholic Americans, products of parochial schools but with no sense of the parish identity that held families and communities together for so many years. She intends to let her seldom-used confirmation name drop but will retain her maiden name. He gives his current address.

Father Greer looks up, taking off his reading glasses. "Your phone?" The man gives his number. "And yours, my dear?" the priest asks, his expression hovering somewhere between bemusement and fatigue. "Very similar to mine," the young man interjects with a boyish grin.

"Would it be unwise to assume you live together?"

"No, that's correct, Father," he says. "You see, we were dating in Pittsburgh and I got a job in Boston and we wanted to be together and we both had to move and rents are so crazy—"

"I k⌐   I can get you a one-bedroom condo next door for only a hundred and eighty thousand clams. But why? Why do you want to be married in St. Patrick's?"

"It's such a beautiful church, Father, reminds me of the first one I went to as a kid," the young woman says. "We're very much in love, and we want a church wedding. It just wouldn't be right to do it any other way."

"Love." Father Greer nods his head wearily. "That's where you are, but will you stay there? Swept off your feet, infatuated. But what if those jobs go out the window? What if a handicapped child comes along? Love gets pretty worn down after a while. You can't live lives by the American principle of substitution—a baby-sitter instead of a mother, toys instead of time—you need a good anchor and it's not love, not money, not sex. It's spiritual; it's about giving. We all want to take. What have you done spiritually to prepare for it? I took six years to prepare for the sacrament I received. Yours is just as holy.

"And you know what, folks—if the truth be told? It's even more demanding."

"Oh, we're preparing in our own way, Father," the young man says, still smiling, undaunted. He is already used to rebuff; he will be a master salesman someday. "We're not doing this for tax breaks or anything like that. Some people do, you know."

"You're preparing in a natural way; you're telling me that living together is all people need to do nowadays. You both had parochial school educations; don't you think you're living in sin?"

"I feel comfortable with it," the young woman responds. "We're really getting used to each other; there won't be any surprises in this marriage, believe me."

"You know, Father, I don't think anything I did today—or last

night—was any different from a person going to church on Sunday,"
the man adds.

"Using yourself as a norm isn't enough," Father Greer responds.
"God's teachings; the Ten Commandments, that's the norm. This
is a sin against purity. Any way you cut it. If you bend that rule,
what's to say you can't bend the rule about the permanence of
marriage? What happens when you don't want to live *that* teaching
anymore?"

"It was a practical arrangement," his fiancée says, with little of
the conviction with which she entered the room a half hour ago.

"I'm a man of the church; I can't not say these things to you,"
Father Greer continues. His voice is now low and gravelly, as it
becomes late at night or when he is enmeshed in an argument he
despairs of winning. "A person can't live a life with selective theology. You are coming to church to testify, and you ask a priest to
testify, that this is a sacramental union. All those people you invited—do you want me to stand up there before them and unite
you in Holy Matrimony with a straight look on my face? They all
know what's up. Is it some formality so you can have pretty organ
music and flowers and your parents can be happy? Is that what it's
about?"

Father Greer pushes himself back from the desk. "Look, if I didn't
care about you, I could just fill out these forms, give you a booklet
you'd never read, and get you out of here in twenty minutes and
we could have a cold drink, put up our feet, and watch the Red
Sox get pounded again. But you see, I have a bad record at this
marrying business. Terrible. I've married a thousand couples and
half of them didn't make it. One from last year is divorced already.
I'm trying to improve my average."

The young man asks what he and his fiancée should be doing to
prepare for their wedding. Father Greer tells them to frequent the
sacraments—go to confession, which both admit they have not done
for years, and attend weekly Mass. "With housing costing what it
does, I can't expect you to move out, but is there any way you could
live apart in the apartment until you're married?" the priest asks.
At his earlier suggestions they had nodded, albeit unconvincingly.
These last words evoke but a blank look of incomprehension.
"Something—I want you to do *something* to prepare for this. How

much time and energy went into finding a caterer, a hall, a band, getting the invitations printed and mailed, the flowers; you probably spent more time on flowers than . . . Okay, here it is: you want to invite Jesus Christ to be at the nuptial union when He hasn't been in your lives. He's a stranger. Is that fair to Him or you to have a stranger at your wedding?"

"But I feel He has been there, Father," the young man says.

"I think you got us all wrong," the young woman adds quickly. "It means a lot to us. We could just go our separate ways—"

"—or get married like this," Father Greer interrupts. "But there's a third way. To be prepared, spiritually prepared, for the most important day in your entire life." It is nearly ten o'clock; Father Greer is exhausted. His eyelids droop so that they seem to push the lower lids down onto his flushed cheeks.

"We'll . . . we'll have to think about it, Father," the young man says with only enough conviction to avoid affronting the priest. "And . . . and maybe come back and see you. Do we have a deal?"

Father Greer says little more as he completes the form. He has made his point; he may act like the Hound of Heaven but does not want to be the Badger of the Boston Archdiocese. "My job isn't to be popular, it's to uphold the truth, and that's not always fun, believe me," he says in parting as he pats them on the back. "Good luck. Think about it; that's all I ask."

And the hundred-thousand-dollar couple goes forth into the balmy Natick night, having come for a routine interview about their church wedding only to find it much more complicated and demanding than they'd bargained for, because of a priest they had not known an hour earlier.

His day over, a Scotch on the rocks in his hand, Father Greer sinks into the lounge chair in his living room. He has functioned within a wide theological range this evening, from utter orthodoxy to compassionate liberalism, and I ask him why he said what he did and what effect he thinks it will have.

"The parish priest has very few chances to talk with people on the periphery. Even fewer times when you have their full attention. People don't come to confession anymore, and we don't have the manpower to do a parish census; you can't go door to door and find people in need or who are lapsed. Ninety percent of people use church as a gas station; they stop in for a fill-up and pull out. Church is a means, not an end. So you do your best with marriage preparation, or any ritual. At baptisms I tell people they are walking out the door with a saint in their arms and ask what they are going to do to care for it. Tonight, with the first couple, what was there to do? Do you harass a sick person, ask them to get up and take a jog? No, you show them understanding and help them get better. How many marriages do we have in the Catholic Church where a person is living with an alcoholic or a person on drugs or mentally ill, someone who abuses the family? What do you say: 'Blessings upon you and go back into that hell of your marriage'? I used to be able to do that in the old days when I had all the answers, but I can't anymore. They call annulments the Catholic divorce. Call it what you like, but you can't condemn people to a rotten life with someone they shouldn't be married to. You've got to look for a way to give them a break.

"But then, the hundred-thousand-dollar couple. Here we had two nice, decent kids. Like a lot of them, they come in thinking they're doing you a favor by being married in the church. They want the old church beauty, but not old church teaching. Their life-style is breezy and easy; they live by polls. The system is the norm; the only stability they have is winning. No mention of the narrow gate here. I had their full attention for those few precious minutes in there. And they are the strong; they have to get a stiff dose, real marching orders. I had to make the most of it without alienating them or scaring them completely. That would never do, to threaten or coerce them. As for what good it does . . . ?"

He takes a long swallow of his drink. "Probably nothing. But that's up to God. Joe Greer did his best."

4

But we are founding an empire, my boy, an empire that
would have made the Caesar's effort look like so much mud—
and peace, real peace, the Peace of Rome.

Yet that institution which seemed so unshakable was really
brittle in the extreme.

A few weeks after I had begun to follow him on his daily rounds,
Father Greer was scheduled for an assignment outside his parish.
We traveled toward Boston on Route 9, the traffic bumper to bumper
and slow, the product of both the normal morning rush hour and
a road crew making preparations to paint a fresh white stripe. Father
Greer, a man who is always punctual for his professional commitments, had left in plenty of time. His radio was tuned, as it customarily is, to WJIB, a station with an "easy listening" format. He
wound through the streets of Brighton, turned onto Commonwealth
Avenue and, as he drove past the low stone wall at 2121 Commonwealth, instinctively turned the radio off.

"Welcome to the Sacred Acre," he said. "It all starts here." The
tone of his voice was that of a man resigned to the mixture of
majesty and madness the Archdiocese of Boston visits upon her men
in the field.

It was Father Greer's morning to say the daily television Mass
from the newly refurbished chapel in the cardinal's residence. (It
had been redone at a cost of $600,000, which not too many Boston
priests considered a justifiable expenditure.) While he was here, he

planned to stop in at St. John's, his old seminary, located on the same grounds. Besides the residence and seminary, the twenty-six-acre archdiocesan complex contains the chancery office, the tribunal, the religious education office, and various other offices of the engineers, lawyers, administrators, and canon lawyers it takes to run America's third-largest diocese, which numbers some 1.8 million Catholics. These offices, these people—well known to a veteran priest like Father Greer—are housed in a half-dozen buildings, but they are places and faces Father Greer has neither cause nor inclination to spontaneously visit or see.

He had carefully read over the instructions sent out for the twenty-eight-minute Mass he was to say. He was to mention no specific names in the Prayers of the Faithful (an FCC rule); keep his homily short, as there was now live organ music at the Mass; and was to be careful not to insert any ad-libbed prayers. The Mass, carried on Channel 25, has a huge following in Boston, including many homebound and ill viewers, from whom four thousand to six thousand letters are received each month.

Father Greer said the Mass flawlessly and, identifying as he tries to do with whatever group is present, pointed to the crucifix behind him as he began his homily. "Some of you are shut in or sick, maybe retired—the better days behind you, you might think. Maybe you don't feel like you're worth much of anything these days. But Our Lord bought you with a very expensive piece of goods—his only Son. Do you think He's going to let you slip out of His sight? Do you sometimes think He's forgotten you, gone on to better things? Not a chance. You're too precious. The Lord will bless you; just talk to Him. He's blessing you right now, and you might not even know it."

There were none of the sophisticated techniques commonly used in the services of popular Protestant television ministers—no huge choir, no congregation, no prefilmed visual effects, no appeal for funds, no invitation to join. The concentration was on the priest and the Mass, the staples of Catholicism.

The Mass over, we began to walk at a leisurely pace along a winding road that leads to the rear of the archdiocesan property. Father Greer pointed to the old library. When he was a seminarian, it was open only two hours a day. "Who needed to do outside reading?" he asked rhetorically. "Like in the army, if it wasn't issued, you didn't need it. But you know what?" he said, his voice taking on a seriousness he seldom allows himself. "We cared. We really wanted to be priests, and whatever that required, we did it." He smiled. "More or less. See that tomb of Cardinal O'Connell? A lot of high shrubs around it; nice landscaping. Best place to grab a butt between classes. A guy in his mid-twenties sneaking a butt; imagine that."

We walked toward a set of buildings whose architecture testifies to the evolving history of St. John's. To our left were staid, elegant French Gothic structures, studded with turrets and graced by great stone staircases that bespeak the European influence prevalent in the American Catholic Church from the nineteenth century—when formal seminary training was instituted—to the early twentieth century. It was an era of quiet, controlled growth, when the Sulpicians, an order founded to train seminarians, educated sufficient numbers of priests to staff Boston's parishes and actually turned away qualified men because there was simply no need for them in the archdiocese. To the right of those venerable buildings was an enormous modern beige brick edifice with monotonous rows of windows. Compared with the lovely excesses of its progenitor, the newer building is altogether functional and unattractive. This is the huge dormitory and office structure begun just as Father Greer was ordained and finished in 1959, when the Catholic Church was strong, mono-lithic, and growing and her best young men could think of no higher calling than the priesthood.

Father Greer paused at the steps of St. William's Hall. He noted he had hesitated much the same way on a September day in 1953. "Didn't like the look of the place much. Drab, grey, quiet. I said to myself, 'Uh, uh. Greer, I don't think you're going to last too long here.' My parents dropped me, my laundry bag, and a suitcase off and I didn't see them until Thanksgiving."

We walked to the second floor and stopped at room 205. It was now a spacious—though unoccupied—room for one seminarian; in Father Greer's day, it housed two. "Two desks, two beds, two chairs and enough room to turn around. If you had a washbasin, you thought you were at the Hilton. Eighty guys on the floor, two showers. It was like Carthage, cold showers and all. No talking, except for a short period after meals. You walked just so. How did I ever get here? Who knows? God's work. I didn't have a lot to say about it. How did I get through? God, again. That's about it; four and a half years later I was a priest."

As I had come to expect from Father Greer over the weeks we had spent together, it was a typically cryptic summary. While he can be expansive as a storyteller, persuasive as a negotiator, and convincing as a preacher, he is not inclined to dwell upon himself. He had told me many times he is a private person, and while this is certainly so, he is also a man who, if asked a question, answers it. But he is not one to volunteer information. I was coming to understand that his reticence was not only the function of his private side, but that either by training or by nature he didn't consider what he did or had done to be of great interest.

And so the facts, fabric, and texture of Father Greer's life had to be gradually pieced together from what he told me, along with what I gathered from friends, family, fellow priests, and parishioners. Most of them, in offering what they did know of Father Joseph Greer (or Joe Greer), would often admit they could speak only of the surface of the man and would not presume to know what really went on inside him.

A vocation to the priesthood was simmering at the back of young Joseph Terrence Greer Jr.'s consciousness throughout his years at Our Lady of Perpetual Mission grade school in the 1940s, as it did for many Catholic schoolchildren of the era. After all, the most prestigious person within the parish—which marked not only the religious but also the social boundaries for most Catholic families of the day—was the priest. And besides being an honored member of the community, he was doing *good*, which was far more important than material success. But young Joe had other things on his mind. For one thing, he was a great athlete—scrappy, fast, alert—and a career chasing fly balls around Fenway Park's left field in a Red Sox uniform seemed equally honorable as a life dedicated to the pursuit of God and the service of mankind.

His Irish immigrant parents, the former Mary Larkin and Joseph Sr., a postman, while good churchgoing Catholics, never pushed the idea of the priesthood, emphasizing instead the need for the education they themselves had not received. Mary especially had visions for her eldest son far beyond the Greers' second-floor apartment in a three-story Roxbury tenement. When young Joe wanted to go to Mission High so he could continue to play sports with his buddies, Mary Greer put him on a bus for Boston College High School, a Catholic school with a superior reputation that regularly sent its graduates on to college.

When he brought home his report cards—one side of which listed mostly As and Bs—Mary Greer would look at the other side first. The mark for "Effort" was more important.

Joe was never an outstanding student, though quick-witted enough to get by with the minimum of outside schoolwork. But socially he was a hit. His dark hair and appealing grin made him a popular date. He liked to drink and went as far with girls as they would allow in those days, how far only his confessor knew. But even as he grew to the age where youthful idealism is often put aside, he continued to take his religion seriously. He never missed Mass; he remained an altar boy when his friends wouldn't be caught dead in a surplice. To him there continued to be something enormously appealing about the priests he knew, but as Joe looked inside himself he wondered whether he could live their life. Yet hard as the thought of giving up the company and pleasures of women might be, there was something about the ideal these priests embodied that would not go away.

If Joe Greer was battling with himself over the path he ought to take, none of his friends had the slightest idea of it. There was nothing at all sanctimonious about him; he was not one of those young men who would attend Mass with bowed head and fervently clasped hands. He would never discuss a sermon, perhaps only offering a comment at its length and how badly he wanted a cigarette by the end of Mass. At Boston College, while studying for a degree in accounting, he became engaged to his steady girlfriend.

One birthday her parents, responding to their daughter's comment that her fiancé had a religious side, gave him as a present *The Quiet Light*, a biography of St. Thomas Aquinas. Aquinas was far from the prototype of a parish priest, but for some reason the book struck a chord. What Joseph read and saw laid out was a quiet but intensely focused life dedicated to God. In his junior year at Boston College,

without telling his friends or even his parents—and certainly not
his fiancée—Joseph Greer took the entrance exam at St. John's.
Accepted or rejected, he didn't want anyone ribbing him for being
that holy.

Three months later—in August 1953—he learned he had been
accepted. His fiancée was as heartbroken as she was astonished when
her Joe explained why he would no longer be seeing her.

St. John's, founded in 1884, had become legendary for the rigorous training it offered as well as for the plentiful numbers of priests
it was then producing for the ever-growing Catholic population of
Boston. In 1911 it had come under archdiocesan control when the
autocratic William Henry Cardinal O'Connell dismissed the Sulpicians and replaced them with a faculty made up of his own priests.
It was O'Connell who began to preach unswerving allegiance to
Rome—a new concept for the young American church—and under
Rome to the archdiocese, in an era when the American hierarchy
was beginning to sense its place in the worldwide church as well as
the power it might wield. O'Connell envisioned St. John's as a
flame to soften, like so much wax, idealistic young men to receive
the sacramental seal of ordination. Its imprint—and their allegiance
to the cardinal—was meant to be deep and sure. The "new" parish
was to be an instrument of the chancery, and its pastor, a courteous
and docile agent. O'Connell's successor and Joseph Greer's first
ordinary, Richard Cardinal Cushing, reinforced O'Connell's strict-
ness and added another, seemingly unreachable goal: he wanted to
be the first Catholic prelate in America to ordain one hundred men
a year.

Such a dream was possible in postwar Boston, the most Catholic
city in the United States, for this was the age of American Catholic
romanticism—a time when Bishop Fulton J. Sheen's television
program was an immense success; when Thomas Merton's *The
Seven Storey Mountain,* an account of his spiritual search and the
Trappist life he chose, was a best-seller; when people crowded into
churches for weekday devotions and packed the pews each Sunday;
when Catholics, no longer poor and struggling immigrants in the
main, were secure in their belief and proud of their unswerving
faith.

The best young men from the area streamed to St. John's, proudly regarded as the West Point of seminaries. In Father Greer's time there were four hundred from Boston. To attain the priesthood they were willing to endure years of harsh discipline and routinized education. Faculty members stood in the hallways and handed out demerits to seminarians not only for smiling or talking, but for walking in an unbecoming way or holding books in a sloppy manner. The seminarians lived all but forty-five minutes of their day in silence, listened to lectures where questions were the sign of apostasy, not an inquiring mind, and visited the library at their peril. Seminarians were taught what was called "the fullness" of their religion through texts by such renowned clerics as Adolphe Tanquerey, who preached dogmatic Roman Catholic theology as the *sine qua non* of spirituality, and Jean-Marie Hervé, whose four-volume scholastic treatise on dogma made selective use of passages from Scripture and the writings of the church fathers to support Rome's doctrines and dismiss all others. Reformers like Calvin, Zwingli, and Luther were cited only to be refuted. Defending the faith was far more important than being able to explain it. Intellectual martial law was in force, and the curriculum—heavy on philosophy, theology, church history, and canon law—was little changed from O'Connell's day.

Nevertheless Joseph Greer and his classmates, looking positively Roman in cassocks, flowing black capes, and birettas, walked contentedly about the grounds under Cushing's proud gaze. They were "Boston," and that was sufficient unto itself, the best and most loyal, proper and provincial crack troops ready to do battle with the evils of the world that waited outside their carefully maintained and controlled compound. Their wood-paneled refectory looked as if it had been plucked from an English boarding school; it was an altogether heady atmosphere for these young men, many of them from humble homes.

"No one thought that we should be treated any other way," Father Greer said as our footsteps resounded in the empty dormitory hallway while we made our way to the crypt, where he had served scores of Masses in preparation for saying his first Mass almost thirty years before. "If you wanted to be a diocesan priest, this is what you did. Means to the end. The only means. You were supposed to cut all ties to old friends, and subtly they even built an invisible wall between you and your family. I was never as close to my family as I was before the seminary, and you know, it's a loss I've grown to regret. They kept drumming it into us that our work here was not only sacred but confidential. You were afraid to say anything to your family, and although I would often go home to West Roxbury to visit, I felt that my parents—God rest their souls—and my brother and sister didn't understand what I was doing. The other future priests did, so you gravitated toward them. They became your family. It was brainwashing to be sure, cutting the umbilical cord; we called it the 'lockup.' We couldn't even be in the room when our parents brought clean laundry once a week. The private good had to suffer for the common good so you could devote yourself entirely to the priesthood, the family of God. At least that's what they told us."

We walked down a set of stairs in the basement of Theology House and into a darkened area. Even though it was a warm summer day outside, it was suddenly cold and damp. Father Greer felt along the wall for a switch. "The crypt," he said, his voice echoing ominously as the lights went on.

Along the walls were identical alcoves, each with an altar, seventeen of them altogether. On a low stone table, in what had obviously been used as the dressing area, was a pile of chasubles, the old fiddleback variety, so named for their shape and stiffness. They were made of lush satin, some frayed, but still in good repair. It was as if the priests, on a certain day years ago, had said their Mass, unvested, and left this part of the church behind.

"In the morning it was like the floor of the New York Stock Exchange," Father Greer said. "All these voices mumbling, bells ringing. Except it was all in Latin, of course. We watched how it was done. When the time came, we wanted to be able to say the perfect Mass."

The seminarians learned when in the course of the Mass to speak *submissa voce*, in a voice only the priest can hear, and when to emote *clara voce*. They were schooled with choreographic precision in when and how to bow, the exact position of fingers and thumbs—together, pointing upward, diagonal, bent, straight—and how far arms should be spread apart at what moment in the Mass. Under

pain of sin, they were to say the Mass in precise Latin, the words
to be uttered without inflection or emphasis. Cardinal O'Connell
had declared, "There is no such thing as the personality . . . of a
parish priest. Personal qualities are subject to change. These are
transient things on which depend nothing of the certainty of the
Catholic faith."

There was to be a sameness about them. In a sense, they were
to be drained of emotion—just as they were to shed any doubt as
to the rightness and fullness of Catholic doctrine—so that only right
reason, a reason formed during the seminary years, would hold
sway. They were to travel over the peaks and through the valleys
of their parishioners' emotional lives—birth, sickness, marriage, the
getting of a job, the loss of a job, a lapse into mental illness, death—
but the priest would have no digressions or lapses himself. The priest
would be neither a husband nor a biological father; he would seek
friendship and whatever intimacy was possible after such rigorous
training only in the company of his fellow priests. Of course, he
would refrain from sexual acts and fight even the thought of such
deeds, having learned and practiced such techniques as "custody of
the eyes" when presented with a potentially sensual person, place,
or thing.

Joseph Greer, although a good and loyal son of St. John's and
most desirous of becoming a priest, didn't quite fit the churchly
mold. He was known as a jock, and a classmate, Father William
Francis, remembered that "He looked a little like a hood, a tough
guy." He was not a particularly distinguished student and was certainly never considered for the upper of the two diocesan tracks,
which led, through advanced studies either at home or in Rome,
to a career in the seminary or chancery and eventually to the hierarchy. Joseph Greer was destined to be an infantryman, a foot
soldier for Christ.

"Joe came off at first impression as maybe a little shallow, a joker,
and definitely a man's man; you could tell he was really put off by
the limp-wristed, faint ones in our class," recalled Edward Roach,
a former priest who is now an executive with Digital Equipment
Corporation. "He used his elbows in basketball, and when he tagged
you in touch football, you knew it. But when we were choosing up
for a game and one of those wimpy guys was left, Joe would always

take him on his side. The ball was snapped and this guy would go wobbling down the sideline. Nobody in their right mind would throw the ball to him, and there was Joe, lofting a sweet little pass to the guy. Of course it bounced off his head. And Joe would go over, toss his arm around the guy's shoulder, and apologize for throwing a bum pass. He had that amazing ability to overcome his dislikes. You never said, 'Greer is a holy guy' or 'Greer is really charitable.' But looking back, you see him better for what he really was. Other guys looked for the status jobs at the sem—not Joe. He was dedicated to the ideal, the idea of moral excellence. He was the kind who would die for a cause. And, as is often the case, a great sense of humor often hides a deep spirituality."

The class, seventy-six strong, was ordained on February 3, 1958, promising Cushing and his successors their unwavering obedience and respect. There was no doubt—it was not even considered an issue, so firm was their confidence in their calling—that ensuing reunions would continue to see them gather as a group, their number diminished only by poor health or death. Certainly there was no thought given to defections from this, the highest calling of Catholic life. Oddly, although they were expected to spend the rest of their lives doing parish work, a good number of them had never spent a single night in a rectory during their training. For that matter, there were few among the faculty who had ever worked in parishes. "It was an amazing system," noted Father Francis. "For years they dressed you like a girl and treated you like a child and then all of a sudden expected you'd be a man."

Father Greer and I completed our tour of the seminary, pausing to look at class pictures in the new main building. After the war, in the early 1940s and 1950s, the faces became smaller and smaller, the shrinkage necessitated by the increasing number of newly ordained priests in each picture. Then, in 1967, the faces started to grow larger, with fewer men within the frame. After 1972 class pictures were discontinued. "And there's the guy who started it all," Father Greer said, pointing to a color photo of the jowly, smiling Pope John XXIII. "Wonder if he had a clue. We sure didn't. Babes in the woods; we went out there thinking the world would never change."

Father Joseph Greer, "the holy oils not yet dry," as they say of newly ordained priests, was sent to his first assignment, St. Joseph's in Quincy. His theology was rigid, his senses anesthetized, and his family and personal life were relegated to their properly insignificant place. He had been perfectly prepared, and he couldn't wait to get at the job. As the junior curate, he was assigned to work with the altar boys, the Catholic Youth Organization, the Ladies' Sodality, the Holy Name Society—and the bowling league. He was expected to say one Mass a day, spend sufficient time in his room or the church or walking about to say his breviary (which, although Latin had been taught at St. John's, was often incomprehensible to him and many of his classmates when it went beyond the familiar, ritual prayers), visit homes and hospitals, take Communion to the sick, hear confessions, assist in a biannual census, conduct classes for converts, and be available for evening consultations. In those days the rectory was the forum for permission—to attend a non-Catholic marriage ceremony, practice the rhythm method of birth control, see a movie "objectionable in part," or read a banned book—as well as the home of the only intermediary many Catholics knew. Courts, police stations, and social workers were for those not of "the faith." Catholics could count on Father if domestic squabbles or drinking tore at the fabric of family life or an errant teenager needed some convincing. "I was overwhelmed," Father Greer said one night as we drove through his old Quincy parish, "not with work, but with bringing Christ down upon the altar at Mass, sitting in a confessional, one person to another, talking about the most intimate things; having men tip their hat to me on the street. Just being called 'Father.' "

Father Greer put in more hours then than he does now, but even allowing for the difference in age, he found it easier. "Nobody criticized you. It was wonderful. We priests had all the answers. And seeing that most of the parishioners at that time didn't have much education, they didn't even know what questions to ask. If they didn't go along with you, you simply said they were going to hell. I condemned more people to hell than I care to remember."

Father Greer was a popular priest, engaging, a good athlete who could mix it up on the sports field with the most agile teenagers. And demanding. The young curate held such great respect for the Mass that if an altar boy came to the sacristy in white socks or tennis shoes, he was not allowed to serve. A serious sin revealed in confession to Father Greer, regardless of the circumstances, would receive a severe penance. Compassion was a foolish concept; discipline was what mattered.

The faint tremors of social unrest in the early sixties were no more than a minor annoyance to Father Greer as he happily lived out the first years of his priesthood. Priests like James Groppi, who was battling school segregation, and the Berrigan brothers, who were antiwar activists—men who presumed to speak from their own consciences and not reflect that of their bishop or provincial—were in his eyes an embarrassment and a scandal. Even the Second Vatican Council, convened by Pope John XXIII, seemed so distant, so theoretical. He was sure the proclamations, about everything from changing the Liturgy to beginning a dialogue with non-Catholic faiths, would soon be gone like so much smoke in the wind— especially in proper and mighty Boston, the bastion of orthodoxy. His archbishop, Cardinal Cushing, likewise waited for these annoyances to pass until one March day in Holy Week, 1966, at a meeting he had called with the pastors of his diocese, Cushing went to the window to witness an astounding sight: a hundred and twenty-five of his own seminarians, carrying placards, were demonstrating against their educational strictures and specifically against their rector, Monsignor Lawrence J. Riley. Henceforth, throughout the archdiocese, the incident would be ominously referred to as "The Trouble," and it marked the beginning of dramatic upheaval and the first significant changes since the seminary's founding.

New courses in human development, psychology, and sociology were introduced as the seminarians were released from their hermetically sealed world with its rigid curriculum. They were allowed to take courses at schools like Harvard and Boston University, members of the Boston Theological Institute that the seminary finally joined. Field education was extended to give a true picture of the priest's work; seminarians actually went to live in rectories. And although they were hardly in the vanguard of the spirit that pervaded so many college campuses in the late 1960s and early 1970s, seminarians began to *talk with* faculty and administration, instead of *being talked to.*

Changes in Liturgy and theology and in the attitudes of a now far better educated Catholic laity pounded on the once-secure psyche of Father Greer. This was coupled with the confusion over the defection of the ever-growing numbers of priests who responded to the more open attitude of the 1960s by leaving the church that had both mothered and smothered them. "It was an awful time to be a priest," Father Greer recalled. "After knowing everything, you knew nothing, didn't know which end was up. We did so many crazy things."

The old structure was crumbling, archdiocesan edicts commanding obedience elicited only indifference, and many priests, feeling the new freedom, acted out their enfranchisement with adolescent glee. Father Greer cleaned out his file drawers and boxes, threw away his seminary notes, his old sermons and commentaries, and his jottings on marriage, sin, and papal infallibility. He stocked his closet with brightly colored shirts, trousers other than the conventional black, and a couple of fashionably tailored sports jackets. He went out for the evening with similarly dressed priest friends, but now it was no longer to a restaurant for early dinner, but to cocktail lounges late at night, hoping no one would recognize them. He drank more than he knew he should. He talked to young women who found him as appealing and engaging as his many parishioners had done over the years. He danced, and the vow of chastity no longer seemed the strict charge to which he'd pledged perpetual fealty. There were stormy nights and foggy mornings. "I wasn't the ugliest guy in the world; sometimes I wish I had been," he recalled. "It might have been easier. I always felt horrible afterwards. I had failed the priesthood, failed myself, and hurt another person. I always wondered what my mother and father thought, looking down from heaven. My mother idolized me so. Sex was a pleasure in those days, but it was a false pleasure. There was no happiness in it for me. I was somehow, somewhere, looking for satisfaction. In all the wrong places. All the wrong ways."

During those troubled years men who had similarly transgressed continued to leave, including those he considered some of the best men in his class. "Only the dross was left, it seemed to me." Other priests defied the entire concept of the diocesan priesthood by specializing themselves out of parish work. Father Greer, confused about his role in a changing church and society but not knowing what else he could possibly want to do, struggled to keep at the work to which he had pledged himself. In the spirit of Vatican II, he joined the archdiocesan Priests' Council and served on the liturgical commission.

His personal and professional lives were beginning to stabilize somewhat just about the time Judge W. Arthur Garrity's order to integrate the Boston public schools came down. Anticipating violence, Humberto Cardinal Medeiros, Cushing's successor, appealed to his priests to ride the school buses to safeguard the passage of black students to white areas. At the time there were a small number of Boston priests fervently committed to civil rights, but Father Greer was not among them. He was serving, as he always had, in an all-white parish, St. Mark's in Dorchester, a section of Boston in what would become the epicenter of integration-related violence. And he still harbored memories from his youth, when blacks and Irish would nightly trade taunts, fists, rocks, and bottles up at Roxbury Crossing.

The integration order was unpopular among white Catholics, but by now Father Greer had learned how to deal with disagreement among the laity. It was equally unpopular with priests, including many of his friends, men he had gone to seminary with and continued to see as golf partners. Joe Greer was no bleeding-heart liberal when in the pulpit and certainly not when in the company of other priests.

"Look, I don't love blacks as much as I love my own Irish people," he recalled one evening as we sat talking. "But God made us all, and He didn't make any garbage. We'd boxed the blacks into Roxbury, and that had to stop. Was I enthusiastic about doing something about it? No. Did I jump into my clerical collar each morning and say, 'Greer lands a punch for equality'? No. I was ordained to help people, and right then, the blacks needed help."

Father Greer was one of the few priests in the entire Dorchester area who responded to the cardinal's plea. "I had started questioning myself, that's all it was. I began to take off the armor of surety and put on the mantle of doubt. Because of my own sinfulness, I could recognize my conservative smugness about social issues, and I couldn't live with it anymore. And I began to see my church more clearly, how we'd been like the people who passed by in the story of the Good Samaritan. We always had an excuse; we didn't take the risk."

His parishioners were not so strangely warmed by the thought of their priest helping blacks to violate an all-white neighborhood that had been preserved as such by decades of commonly accepted prejudice. Some of his fellow priests were also not pleased as Father Greer rode into South Boston on those charged mornings. The incoming buses were pelted with rocks and splattered with garbage. One kindly-looking older lady held a rosary in one hand and greeted the buses with the obscenely extended middle finger of the other. Once within closer range, Father Greer was regularly spat upon. At a restaurant in Dorchester one evening, following a television appearance in which he had advocated calm, an enraged waitress threw a salad in his face. Threatening and abusive calls were daily occurrences at the rectory, and the bitterness spilled over to other church activities. Only after he had finally found enough money for hockey nets and convinced the public works department to stripe the churchyard did Father Greer discover the full measure of his people's hate. Within two days the nets were torn apart, the adhesive striping peeled from the concrete.

Father Greer's reward for adroitly handling one touchy job was to be given another, this time as pastor of St. Joseph's in Hyde Park, a once-white parish in the process of being integrated. Traditionally, pastors were assigned on a strict seniority basis. At the time they could expect their first pastorate twenty-six years after ordination. But when the cardinal's staff looked at the growing number of potential tinderbox parishes and then at the qualifications of the men available—their degree of racial enlightenment, mental health, and physical stamina—they began to reach down to more junior men to fill the posts. Father Greer had been ordained nineteen years before; his appointment made him one of the youngest pastors in Boston's recent past. He served at St. Joseph's for seven years before coming to St. Patrick's.

Father Greer's years of upheaval had paralleled the upheaval in his church, but he was still a functioning priest. "Why did I make it through? Why am I not bitter, like so many of the guys who left and even a lot who are still in? Not because I'm such a wonderful human being, believe me." He looked through his rearview mirror as we left the archdiocesan grounds.

"A little bit of luck and a lot of God's grace, that's why."

5

Yet all the same our way isn't the way of the world. You can't go offering the truth to human beings as though it were a sort of insurance policy, or a dose of the salts.

If his own disposition and history are any guide, Father Greer is not destined to become an inspirational leader seen on videotapes or the author of books advising people how to lead fuller inner lives. Nor does he any have special insights to share with fellow clergy on how to reform their religious institutions. Unlike the Natick rabbi Harold Kushner, a popular speaker and author of the best-selling *When Bad Things Happen to Good People*, Father Greer is unknown outside his local area. Unlike such Catholic priests as Gustavo Gutierrez and Leonardo Boff, whose liberation theology aims to revolutionize a church they feel has lost its compassion and vision, Father Greer has nothing especially new to say about the form and substance of the Catholic Church. Literally hundreds of books pour out each year from the presses telling clergy how they can better serve their congregations, improve their services, sacraments, homilies, and visits, and manage their property, funds, and time more effectively. Father Greer would laugh at the thought that he could add anything about how to be a better priest, pastor, or person. In fact, he would be loath to add to the prodigious outpouring of so many others who are eager to have their voices heard and their faces seen.

While hardly a man unwilling to change or respond to the movement of his church, Father Greer does not think of himself as being *au courant,* nor does he have the desire to be so. He maintains that his theology could be summarized in the Beatitudes—those supplications to thirst after justice, be poor in spirit, meek, merciful, pure in heart, a peacemaker, righteous, and willing to be persecuted when in pursuit of that righteousness. "What else is there to say? The job is to live them. Nothing new or trendy about that." He is not at home with many of the words that currently fuel the new vision of the priesthood. *Empowerment. Facilitate. Collaborative ministry. Process.* These terms are not within his lexicon and actually irritate him.

Had he saved his thirty years of desk calendars, he would find that his early years of the priesthood showed a heavy emphasis on the religious side of the priesthood—from religious instruction to a plethora of rituals—the middle years, during the late 1960s and 1970s, more of the temporal, and the present years a heavy measure of both.

He was made aware during his seminary training that he would have to perform diverse temporal and religious tasks, with the accent decidedly on the religious. But the church's more aggressive recent posture on social justice, coupled with the declining number of priests, has placed a far greater burden on the shoulders of those who have stayed in harness. Where once many pastors were content to be figureheads in the community, influencing by mandate or mere presence, they are now asked to be community leaders who actively participate. In the spiritual realm, it is no longer enough to go through the rituals of Mass or matrimony or burial year after year with the same flatly intoned Latin words. Today's priests are expected to make those rituals new and meaningful each time.

Taking a closer look at Father Greer's temporal work in the Natick community, it becomes clear that his style and technique owe much to the fact that he was born and raised a Boston Irishman. The greater Boston area is a major metropolis, but one with many definable neighborhoods and strong religious and ethnic predispositions. It is predominantly Catholic and Irish. It is a city that can be, as politicians would say, "worked," because it is still ethnically, religiously, and culturally stratified. A person's neighborhood, be it Chelsea or Cambridge or Everett or Brockton or Natick—and often a given *part* of that neighborhood—still says something about that person, perhaps gives him or her a certain slant on the world. Catholic parishes—though surely not the centers of people's lives in the same way they were when Father Greer was growing up— have enormous spheres of influence. Many of Boston's powerful are parishioners—if only in name—somewhere. The interlocking sectors of churches, schools, neighborhoods, political offices, and the huge city and state government bureaucracies provide an enticing, but often ultimately solvable, puzzle for those audacious enough to play.

All those days—from the Roxbury triple-decker on through Boston College and the seminary and five parishes—taught Joseph Greer, an alert, instinctive student of human nature as well as power politics, when to write a letter to a high-ranking official and when to talk to the worker who actually can get the job done. When to wear the collar and when presuming upon clerical privilege would work to his disadvantage. When a member of the so-called "Irish Mafia" should be consulted or his own Boston College days or Catholicity proclaimed. When to mention the sheer number of his parishioners to someone in an elected office to whom their votes might be crucial. He has had meetings with Senator Edward Kennedy and former Speaker of the House John McCormack, as well as all the state representatives and senators who represented his various parishes. He knows not to call out for favors—or apply pressure—unless he has a good chance of succeeding.

It is a measure of his influence and tact that when "Father Greer of St. Patrick's" is on the phone to a bureaucrat or politician, the call is usually taken or quickly returned.

While he is adept with the phone and certainly not shy about going to government offices, Father Greer, as he did in his former parishes, continues to make it a point to be a visible presence in Natick. Often he takes a three- or four-mile walk through the parish, stopping on the street to talk with a person who hasn't been in church lately or one, regardless of religious affiliation, whom he knows has had some personal tragedy or is currently in need. He knows the meter maid, store owners, town employees, a large number of the children, the recent winners of Megabucks legal gambling, and the retarded man who walks his dog and threatens, as he does when he sees the priest, to bring it into church one day. "Not that dog!" Father Greer exclaims with fresh indignation each time. "A Protestant if I ever saw one!"

Like other, better-known Boston pols, he moves in many worlds, knows where power and wealth reside and how to get things done, from obtaining free sports tickets to making sure St. Patrick's is the first of the Natick churches to have its parking lot plowed on snowy Sunday mornings. And because of his stature as the pastor of one of the largest churches in the area—but as much or more because of his personal charm—many groups and individuals, both Catholic and non-Catholic, ask him to bless their wedding, dance, party, or dedication with his presence. He is constantly being asked to dinner by parishioners and admits to a habit of "ecclesiastical lying" to excuse himself, making use of whatever extenuating circumstance (an unpredictable schedule, a wake, a heavy counseling load) comes to mind. It is not only that he is weary of nervous wives preparing a meal as if he were visiting royalty, but those who invite him tend to be those in the upper social strata of the parish and not those who, being of lesser means, might be more in need of his attention. He also realizes there is a certain status attached to having the pastor to the house, and he does not want to be a partner in such intraparish competition.

And yet when the son of one of his parishioners was about to open a new White Hen Pantry convenience store and the woman wanted it blessed, Father Greer obliged, giving a touching blessing that included a petition that the employees would be safe—as such twenty-four-hour stores are often prey to robbers. He goes along with many such requests, handling with equanimity the sublime and the ridiculous, seldom staying for more than half an hour at any social event.

But when he feels his presence is being used to sanction something he does not believe in, he is not a man to mask his sentiments. Shortly after he came to St. Patrick's, he was invited to speak at a "fund-raiser for Ireland" that was being promoted and attended by some of his most prominent parishioners. By the tenor of the comments at the bar, he quickly realized he was at a clandestine IRA rally. When a fellow priest fervently and theologically promoted the killing of Protestants in Ireland as God's will, Father Greer bluntly told the priest he did not look like Moses and that the Ten Commandments—including the fifth, " 'Thou shalt not kill,' Father,"—were in effect for everyone. And he walked out.

It is a rare week that does not see Father Greer in the Natick town hall, just up East Central Street from St. Patrick's. It might be to push through plans for the clubhouse renovation, to attend a meeting on affordable housing, to remind the town that it had better lean a little harder on the MBTA to do something about the St. Patrick's parking lot, or to see Fred Conley, the town administrator, about the repairing of a cracked sidewalk in front of the convent on which one of the retired nuns recently tripped.

A Jesuit for nine years, Conley, who has certainly dealt with his share of those devoted to God's service, is a great admirer of Father Greer, calling him by far the most concerned clergyman in Natick. "When he walks in here, he doesn't play clerical games with you," Conley said. "He can be very tough when he's negotiating, but you know he's being tough in order to accomplish something for other people. It's never a personal battle with him. Although he's proud and feisty, he really doesn't have the kind of ego that demands that he win. He just stays with the issue, doesn't demean or overly praise, and he has always done his homework. He's willing to do the ordinary jobs, the mundane, the time-consuming. He saw people staggering up the steps at St. Patrick's, and he whipped through plans for an elevator for the handicapped before we could even turn around. He gets the permits when he feels he has to, and he works around them when he can. He could have had a lot of careers, I'm sure, but he would have made a superior ward heeler.

"The St. Patrick's parking lot is a perfect illustration of what he's about. Joe Greer is not going to be a patsy. If the MBTA commuters are using it, the authority is going to maintain it and pay for the privilege. He's willing to use brinkmanship—like locking out the cars one morning—to get their attention and mine, but it's never a power struggle. It's a way of running a parish well, utilizing the resources, and Joe Greer is a great resource manager. He's doing it for his people. And people like him; that's a big plus. Look, three of the four members of the town finance committee are his parishioners. He's smart enough to never try to strong-arm anyone, but it's pretty clear what he wants. He's willing to attend those interminable meetings, to say something when it makes sense and be quiet when that will work.

"In the seminary, we had a saying that we'd come out with after we'd been up to our eyeballs in Marcel or some heady existential discussion. 'After all the talk, you got to be able to make sandwiches.' In city government, a lot of people come in with great theories that they are not willing to follow through on. Joe Greer can make sandwiches."

I was coming to know Father Greer in his various public roles, and the adroitness with which he handled them amazed me repeatedly. With time it became clear that some of the same characteristics that made him an effective administrator and public figure also came into play in his religious duties. He maintained his unerring ability to see the nature of the task at hand clearly and to size up his audience, even in a sense to perceive himself from their point of view, so that while neither acting as a clerical chameleon nor pandering to what people might like to hear from him (the hundred-thousand-dollar couple being a perfect example), more often than not he succeeded in discharging his obligations wisely.

On Sundays, it is not extraordinary for Father Greer to say three Masses. One late-summer Sunday when I was with him he had to say four: the first in the early morning at St. Patrick's, another at midmorning at a Natick senior citizens' residence, the third at noon at a neighboring parish, and the last in the afternoon at St. Patrick's. He tried to reshape his homily for each audience.

He was up at 5:30, the usual hour of his Sunday rising, and as soon as he had showered and shaved, began his day by rereading of the day's Gospel, the familiar parable of the sower and the seed. He had made notes for his sermons during the four or five times he had read the Sunday Gospel in the days leading up to the weekend, letting the passage bestir his mind. But when he mounted the pulpit he carried nothing.

For the morning St. Patrick's congregation, he began on a personal note: "When I was a boy, I liked the movies, cowboy movies especially. Good guys with the white hats on the white horses, the bad guys with the black hats and dirty clothes—and of course, those black horses for them. Oh, it was so wonderful to know exactly what was what. That's the way I left the seminary; I knew it all. Then, bingo, eighteen of my classmates left the priesthood. Wait a minute, these were the guys in the white hats! You know what we found out? We, the wheat, weren't perfect at all. . . ."

At Cedar Garden, the retirement home: "What if God plucked you out the first time you failed? Can you think back to all those things you did years and years ago that make you blush today? What if he would have said, 'Sorry, Rita, sorry, Joe, you're a weed for sure and into the fire you go.' Not many of us would have made it to be together this Sunday morning, would we? What if God judged us as quickly as we judge each other? Are we loving each other the way he loved us? Hey, this looks like a pretty pious bunch, but I'm squinting and I don't see any halos out there yet . . ." Laughter.

At St. Linus, a neighboring church whose pastor had fallen down his cluttered stairway and broken some ribs and where the windows of the home of a Vietnamese family who had recently moved into the parish had been shattered during the past week: "We knew it all—the Protestants were the weeds and they went to hell and the Catholics were the wheat and we went to heaven. And to be an Irish Catholic! Well, that was the tallest, fullest stalk, of course. So it came to prom time, and I asked my father to use the car and he asked who I was taking and I proudly answered, 'Grace Tartaglia! She's beautiful, Pop!' My father, by the way, thought that God spoke with a brogue. 'An Italian! You're going to the prom with an Italian! No way!'

"We've come a long way—we even have services with the Protestants now and Italians are marrying Irish all over the place and raising some fine families. But where are the weeds in our lives today? Who are we looking down on? Are we loving our neighbor as ourselves or are we all looking around to pull up anything that looks like it might be a weed? Let God do that; he knows the plant life a lot better than you and I. Just try to get along. Remember when somebody didn't like you for what you were? Doesn't everybody in here have a story on that account? I can tell you some from my days at Roxbury Crossing that would turn your hair white. Those of you with hair, that is . . ." Laughter.

The afternoon Mass, at 5:30 P.M., is the one Father Greer and the other priests at St. Patrick's dread. It is at the end of their busiest day; by this time they have said several Masses, overseen a number of collections, greeted the people after each Mass, perhaps performed a baptism, and dealt with a string of people who come to church on Sunday and want to transact their parish business at the rectory on the same trip. And, as Father Greer had said of the 5:30 congregants, "It's the end of their day, too; maybe they've been to the beach, out on the boat; they want a performance. They expect you to change water into wine up there."

Father Greer read the parable of the sower for the fourth time. His voice was flat and fatigued, and the lines came out sing-songy, the emphasis seemingly placed on all the wrong words. "So how do you treat the weeds in your lives? What about this church of ours; how are we doing? The old days were great, right? I'd babble up here for a half an hour in Latin, tip my biretta, and off I'd go. Then that plump little pope, John XXIII, changed it all. The church began to identify with the people. We began to admit that we had some weeds. All the sureness went, and with it went a lot of people, too. Look, after the day I've had I'm about to go out the window myself." Laughter.

"What is the Scripture saying to us? Love one another. What is the church saying? It's hard to tell a weed from a sprout. Love one another, that's all. That's all any of us can do."

On this Sunday Father Greer's day did not end with the 5:30 Mass. He was the priest on duty and had to be available for any emergency calls. In what is getting to be a common practice in Catholic parishes, Father Greer took along an electronic beeper in case he had to be summoned during dinner at a nearby restaurant. As he sat in a sport shirt and slacks, sipping his Manhattan in a booth at Callahan's, a popular local steak house, he seemed to shrink before my eyes. It had nothing to do with posture; he was simply no longer the imposing man in black striding into a sacristy to vest or standing in the pulpit in flowing white vestments talking before hundreds of people about a sower and his seeds. Joe Greer now seemed a quite ordinary man slouched over his cocktail, scanning a menu that he was not really reading—because he orders New York sirloin every time. He looked tired, but equally he looked relieved, the relief of a man who has worn a uniform all day long and is finally able to take it off.

I had recently been with Father Greer during many of those on-duty hours, as he joined young couples in marriage and older ones also, with some years and children behind them. I had listened to how he always fashioned a service that mixed love and religion ("Like the song says, love isn't love until you give it away; look at that cross—that's giving it away") with his innate sense of humor, always concluding the ceremony with some version of his customary parting dictum ("Now, I want you to say three Hail Marys; let's get this marriage started off on the right foot—with a little penance").

I had watched him bless the sick and bury the dead and somehow impart something if not always profound, at least memorable and personal each time. But I learned that in a priest's life there are rituals for which he feels unprepared, that no matter what depth of experience or spirituality he might possess, he senses himself woefully inadequate to the moment.

Father Greer parked his car a good distance from the gathering of some thirty people, most in their mid-twenties, who were standing in the shade of a huge oak tree. That morning, he seemed not to want to get out of the car. "Oh, boy," were the only words he uttered.

Father Greer unfolded a purple stole and draped it over his shoulders. He walked slowly toward the small group of people, who, as they spread out to greet him, left a narrow open space in their midst. On the well-tended grass was a tiny white coffin. Father Greer knew none of the mourners, but it was not difficult for him to recognize the parents. The husband, chin on his chest, arms limply at his sides, stood beside his wife, whose normally trim figure was still swollen from the pregnancy. She was dressed in a fine rust-colored silk suit, perhaps her going-home outfit or the one chosen for the baptism. After shaking their hands in condolence, Father Greer learned that it was the first child, a girl. She had lived only twelve hours.

He proceeded to the opposite side of the casket and intoned the specified burial prayers. As he asked for a moment's pause for reflection and prayer, he bowed his head. He had buried the child properly, done his duty, and now, and now . . .

He remained in place for perhaps a minute and a half, trying to think what he might say. And nothing came into his mind that made the least sense, nothing that might somehow help the young couple. Were they angry with God for doing this? Had they been churchgoers; what was their faith like? What did the husband do for a living?

Not knowing what else to do, Father Greer made the sign of the cross and others of the gathering did likewise. The priest moved from his side of the casket to theirs. Eyes filled with pain fixed on the man who was somehow supposed to bring aid and comfort to this impossible moment.

"Why do these things happen?" he asked rhetorically. "I don't have an idea. I wish I did. Why did God call her? We just don't know His mind."

Father Greer's voice was not brimming with compassion; it was not especially sad. There was more a certain puzzlement in his tone. "Why does he call any of us to do what we do? Why did he call me to be a priest? I'll have to ask Him, we'll all have to ask Him when we get up there. I try talking to Him now and again, but He's not the best conversationalist, you know."

A few of the mourners mustered small smiles.

"But you know something? Little Katie Ann *is* in heaven. We know that. That's the beauty of it. Some of us have to wait ninety years to get there. She only had to wait one day. Not even a day." The young mother's face brightened ever so slightly; she looked down at the coffin. "Up there in heaven, Katie Ann, nice and comfortable; she doesn't have to worry about this humidity and the lousy flies down here." The woman smiled broadly; fresh tears streamed down her cheeks.

"No, she doesn't, Father; she was so sick," the young mother said. "She wouldn't have been comfortable at all. Thank you, thank you from the bottom of my heart, Father—Father—"

"Greer."

Rituals such as this one, while charged with meaning for the participants, can readily become routine to a priest, a man like Father Greer who has seen so much grace and tragedy arbitrarily commingled during thirty years in the priesthood. Father Greer admits he must constantly guard against ordinariness. He has said over ten thousand Masses in his life and sometimes, while on the altar, cannot, for example, remember if he has said the words of consecration. Weddings, so momentous for the couple, are often grueling ceremonies for the modern-day priest like Father Greer, who rarely knows the couple well and yet is expected to exude a certain amount of excitement. "And they beg you to come to the reception, where you're supposed to sit there like a potted plant. Everybody is on their best behavior and you can tell they're just waiting for you to leave so they can really have a good time." He often has no more than briefly met the parents of the children he baptizes, and he has officiated at hundreds of wakes where he has looked upon the still, fixed face for the first and final time.

And yet, at least during the months I spent with him, it was a rare Liturgy when Father Greer did not appear to be personally involved with the words he was saying, the people before him. I distinctly remember one Mass in particular when he was having an off day. His face was disturbingly lifeless, the phrases came out wooden and rote. It was chilling to see Father Greer without a shred of inspiration, without whatever that power is that transforms him.

One autumn night after dinner at the rectory, when Father Greer was on duty and staying in, I asked him to give me a profile, his view, of the ideal Catholic pastor today.

Uncharacteristically, he was quick—and somewhat lengthy—in his reply. "He is one who reflects Vatican II totally—that is, preaching the Good News and building community among his people— he is accepted by one hundred percent of his parish, spiritually deep, intellectually high, and overflowing with charity. Notice that I say nothing about his administrative abilities. A pastor is the shepherd of sheep; he shouldn't get wrapped up in building the stalls."

He offered an answer to what he sensed might be the next question. "And how do I measure up? Not too well, really. I'm a middle-of-the-road pastor. I sow some good seed and some bad seed. I celebrate the Liturgy well, I think, and preach adequately, but I don't read enough. Ask me about medical ethics, and I don't know beans. I'm not always as good as I could be in counseling because

I have a short fuse. I put people in a time box, fifty minutes tops, and if they spill over, I'm impatient. The other day a lady with an eighteen-year-old alcoholic daughter was evading the issue when I told her she had to set up some rules in her house. She kept going on; she wasn't listening. I looked down at my watch, saw I still had at least ten minutes before Mass, but I lied right to her face and said I had to go right then. And when people don't understand me or do what I think is best, I can be sarcastic; I have a quick tongue and want to use it.

"Emotionally—well, I don't know. I think if I were more emotionally open, it would deepen my prayer life—the more open you are to human beings, the more open you are to God—but I know I have to keep a rein on my emotions. Like burying that baby; if I let my emotions in, I wouldn't be able to function; I couldn't stand the strain day in and day out. Tragedies are so common in my life that in a way they don't become particular, and there is a downside to that. When you stop crying, you close down a part of yourself.

"Let me think about this: when was the last time I was emotionally involved in a funeral? It was when a thirteen-year-old altar boy shot himself in the head. Had to be ten years ago. I said the funeral dry-eyed. Went through a whole day of work. And that night at dinner, I got up from the table and had to throw up.

"Spiritually, I try, but I'd like to be much holier than I am. My biggest problem when I sit down and try to meditate, I'm reflecting with my head, not with my heart. That's not really the best way, intellectualizing. That's not what faith is about, figuring out some formula, some way at it. It's giving in.

"But—and not that I want to stand before God with this excuse— I have so much stuff buzzing around in my head, it's hard to empty it out so God can be let in. Parishioners are donating an average of six bucks a week, three times what it was when I got here; the church exterior is repointed, the lower church will be renovated, the rectory fixed up, the house for the homeless done over; that kind of stuff I do pretty well. I just hope there's something happening in the church, that people's lives are being changed. But who knows about that? I constantly complain that being a pastor is one continuous flogging, which is true. But somehow I know I could do this a lot better. There is a fine line between burnout and full responsibility, and I need to get closer to the line."

6

Last night I became intensely aware of this presence and suddenly caught myself turning my head toward some imaginary listener, with a longing to cry that shamed me.

Father Greer was never one to say much about his disease, except, when asked, to name it, then at times to go on to describe it—although not always with scientific accuracy—and to note that he was being treated at the New England Medical Center, which he described variously as "a renowned institution" or "a first-class place." Perhaps, depending on who asked him, he might point out the date of his next appointment, mentioning it in much the same manner as he would any of the commitments he must schedule in advance.

His work remained in the foreground, the disease in the background, and even Fathers Mullaney and Rossi, who live with him, and the parish secretary, Janet Hamilton, who has known him even longer, found they were left with more questions than answers about the mental and physical state of the pastor.

As Father Greer was a patient diagnosed with a disease with no known cure and undoubtedly fighting an internal battle whose intensity could only be surmised, his staff at St. Patrick's continually wondered how this "iron man" they had come to know was facing the issue of his own mortality. Soon after the diagnosis of multiple myeloma, there had been thought of relieving him of at least one of his responsibilities, the once- and twice-weekly rounds at Leonard Morse Hospital. Father Greer could easily have asked his associates to fill in or simply told the hospital or chancery that he was at risk because of the lowered immunity that myeloma produces and that made him a ready target for infection.

Other priests, after thirty years of hospital rounds, might have found such tours grueling and repetitive and would have been happy to have an excuse, but Father Greer did not seek to be relieved. "You see real changes going on: people coming back to the sacraments, reconciling themselves with God when they know that their time is limited, receiving the grace of conversion," he explained to me after one of the dozens of trips we made to Leonard Morse. "Believe me, after all the uncertainties of parish life, the seeming lack of progress, it can be very heartening; people on the ward can put you on cloud nine. Or, they can drain you. But I was never one to go on my emotions; besides, it's part of my job. I'm still the pastor; I have to set an example. We're still short of priests; I have to do my share."

Father Greer's hospital visits always begin with a trip to the lower church tabernacle, where consecrated hosts are reserved. These tiny wafers have, according to Catholic doctrine, been transformed into the body of Christ at a Mass and are held in readiness for sick calls. Father Greer places some hosts in a pyx, then tucks the metal case— the size of a woman's thick compact—into his inner coat pocket. On his way out of church, he kneels at the altar railing and spends a few minutes in silence. He rarely bows his head at such moments, instead looks directly at the tabernacle or the crucifix behind it. His face is attentive and alert rather than contemplative.

"Want to keep Jesus comfortable," he said one afternoon, patting his chest where the pyx rests, "and give him a smooth ride over. He's a good friend."

At the hospital, he checks off the names of patients listed as Catholic on the fifth floor, the floor for which St. Patrick's has responsibility. He notes only those in rooms below 520. Those above 520 are in the psychiatric ward, where, unlike his assigned patients— most of whom are elderly—the residents are usually young. Most are in as a result of drug or alcohol abuse, others because of suicide attempts or mental breakdowns. Because these patients are already in some form of therapy, it is hospital policy that clergy refrain from visiting them so as not to interfere with their program.

With a wave of his hand to the nurses on duty, a comment about current events ("What do you mean, Oliver North is the anti-Christ?" he might say to the head nurse. "Got your socks on a little too tight today?"), Father Greer is off on his rounds. The weather, the pope, the cardinal, a sports team, or current local news might serve as equally good material. He usually visits ten to fifteen patients, which takes an hour to an hour and a half.

To make hospital calls with Father Greer, I found, was to witness a wonderful clerical adroitness that marvelously incorporated bedside humor, a passing but instant and somehow on-target sensitivity, and a natural sacramental presence. A man in intensive care, his voiceless throat swathed with bandages from a cancer operation, scrawled, "Not sure I'm qualified" in response to Father Greer's offer of the Eucharist, indicating he wasn't in the state of grace. "That guy up there understands you better than you know yourself. Don't worry about the details. Let's say an Act of Contrition together because the Good Lord wants to be here with you right now."

As operating room attendants stood by, he bent over a gurney holding a woman about to go into surgery. Her left leg was a stump, the result of diabetes and poor circulation. A bulging catheter in her right arm told of a history of dialysis. She had a life-threatening bowel impaction. "Now, don't worry about this, Genevive—can I call you Jenny? Jenny, are you sorry for all your sins?" The oxygen tubes in her nose gave the words the woman uttered the quality of being called out from deep inside a cave. "I'm sorry. I'm sorry for everything."

"I know you are, honey," he said. "Let's not worry too much about that," he added as he quickly anointed her with holy oil. "Had the sacrament myself about a year ago, and look at me, still walking around. It's just something to help you along. Oh, I see by your address you're over in St. Joseph's, Father Burckhart's parish. We did time in Norwood together; is he still as ugly as ever?" Father Greer ended his visit with a soothing, if hardly ecclesiastical, "Atta girl," as he patted her arm, waxen, crusted, and bruised from injections.

He realizes the weight his visit brings to a hospital room, the fact that he can as easily be viewed as the Angel of Death as the bearer of spiritual refreshment. "Every person has a reason to refuse you—

might have been hurt or scared by a priest. It's amazing, the stories I've heard of what guilt and shame priests have heaped on to people's shoulders at one time in their life. People don't forget; it haunts them. Or else their faith may be dried up, and on top of that they're sure the doctors aren't telling them everything and you've been sent there ten minutes before they're going to die. They don't need two prophets of doom. When a person is sick and sees a priest, they see DEATH printed in big letters on his forehead. I try to eliminate that. They don't need you coming in there with a long face like your brother is an undertaker and you have a little form for them to sign. The person is depressed. I was depressed when I was lying there. I learned a lot being on the other side. So I try not to act too heavy. They need to laugh or smile as much as they need anything right then."

At a room posted with a PROTECTIVE CARE sign warning visitors to wear masks, Father Greer walked in without one. While such masks protect both the patient and the visitor, Father Greer feels that with a mask he dramatizes the illness and, more than the doctors and nurses who enter, *is* the Angel of Death. With his face exposed, he at least has some chance to reach the patient. This patient, a man in his sixties with pneumonia, was convinced he was sicker than anyone would admit to him. Father Greer sprinkled the room with holy water while intoning a prayer and then opened the pyx. The man's eyes filled with tears as the Host neared his lips. "Get rid of those tears or I'll give you a punch in the trunks," was Father Greer's retort. "I was in here a year and a half ago. Cancer—me, the guy in the white hat. Had the last sacraments and all. You'll be up dancing a jig with the missus in a couple of weeks. Let's see a smile. And give the Lord thanks for keeping you in the ball game for a few more innings. We all can get knocked out of the box any time."

So often, because many of the patients at Leonard Morse are elderly and frequently in advanced states of mental deterioration, Father Greer is visiting patients who do not even know he is there. He does not remain long in the rooms of those whose eyes are closed in sleep or open in a dazed consciousness, but he will always say a few words and recite a prayer, even though for the most part he gets no response. "You never know how much they know," he told me, "and besides, I'm not hurting them by jumping in there for a few minutes."

On one such call, to a eighty-five-year-old woman who had been unresponsive to his visits for weeks and who was expected to die shortly, Father Greer began with some comment about the weather. "Okay, not talking to me today, I see. So let me say a little prayer here, my dear, if I might, before I move on."

As he took the prayer book out of his pocket, the woman's right hand moved off the smooth sheet, and by the time he found the proper prayer, the hand was suspended in midair, as if held by a puppeteer's string.

"The Lord is my light and my salvation;
"Whom shall I fear?
"The Lord is my life's refuge;
"Of whom should I be afraid?"

Her hand moved toward her face and then reversed direction, passing slowly down over her sunken chest. The hand wavered ever so slightly to the left.

"One thing I ask of the Lord;
"This I seek:
"To dwell in the house of the Lord
"All the days of my life,
"That I may gaze on the loveliness of the Lord
"And contemplate his temple."

The hand moved right. And then came to rest on her chest. She had made the Sign of the Cross.

But then there are the days when things do not go well. The teenage girl whose icy stare was her only response as the priest tried to engage her in conversation. The disoriented man who screamed at the priest for waking him. The depressed woman whose complaints he had heard week after week: the nurses don't care, the doctors are treating her for the wrong disease, her family has aban-doned her.

But so often, in the midst of even such draining days as these, there will be a moment that lifts him. A simple thank-you for bringing Communion. "I needed that," an elderly woman said, her eyes closing as if she had tasted a wonderful morsel of food.

"We all need it," he responded as he left the room, the last on his list.

We walked toward the hospital lobby one afternoon, and Father Greer hesitated at the open doors of the chapel. "Concelebrated Mass here once," he said, at once expressionless and somewhat amused by the memory. "Last Easter. In a wheelchair."

Because he had such a wide circle of friends from thirty years of being in the priesthood, Father Greer's hospital calls were not limited to Leonard Morse. There were people like Eddie McDermott to see. McDermott occupied a special place in Father Greer's heart because of that glorious year they teamed up and won the member/clergy golf tournament at the Wampatuck Country Club in Canton. Father Greer had tried to get over to the hospital in Norwood earlier but because of a hectic week that saw the bids come in on the lower church renovation, the MBTA begin to move on the parking lot, and an act of vandalism (potted flowers stuffed into the holy water fonts) that made him decide to close the church immediately after the morning Masses, he had been prevented from doing so. When he arrived late one afternoon it was to find that McDermott had died a few hours before.

His memory of McDermott was as more of a friend with a level backstroke and a picture-perfect follow-through than as a soul in distress who had needed his ministrations. "Let's just hope he's not in a sand trap up there," he said, eliciting a healthy laugh from the nurse on McDermott's floor.

But it would be naïve to assume that Father Greer's visits to sick friends are solely those of some sort of clerical glad-hander out to provide a psychological boost and a chuckle. This became evident in a visit to a man Father Greer knew through his business connections with St. Patrick's. The priest had recommended his services to other pastors, thus significantly increasing his business.

The man had suffered a heart attack, and Father Greer found him in the cardiac care unit, intravenous tubes in both arms, oxygen tube in his nose, a heart monitor at his bedside.

"You bum. You were supposed to take me to lunch. You'd do anything to get out of picking up a check," Father Greer began.

"Next week, the week after. We'll make a date. You know what's the worst thing in here? I need a cigarette."

"Cigarette?"

"Four packs a day. Doesn't go away easy."

"I know. I came in from jogging when I was down in Georgia on vacation a couple years back and almost passed out. I was doing two packs and six or eight cigars. I quit. Cold turkey."

"I can't do that. But when I get out of here in a couple days—"

"Couple days? The Good Lord took seven. What's your hurry? What's this I hear you won't see the hospital chaplain? Want the guy to lose his job?"

"Well, you know how I am. Couple days and I'll be out. What's the big deal? I'm not that sick."

"Unless I'm terribly mistaken, this is the CCU. That stands for cardiac care unit—you know, intensive care for faulty tickers."

"Okay, okay. When I get out. I'm going to change."

"But here you are. I'd like to say a few prayers and like the Lord touched you—he gave me a good whack too—I'd like to touch you in another way." Father Greer opened a small book that had been virtually concealed in his palm.

"O Lord, hear my prayer
"And let my cry come to you
"Hide not your face from me
"In the day of my distress.
"Incline your ear to me;
"In the day when I call, answer me speedily.

"He has broken down my strength in the way;
"He has cut short my days.
"I say: O my God,
"Take me not hence in the midst of my days;
"Through all generations your years endure."

"Something else, my friend, something we call the Sacrament of the Sick these days. I'd like to anoint you and give you the blessing—"

"Just in case. Right, Father?"

"No just in case. Just because its good to have God present for you in a way that the church has used for centuries; to receive a sacrament."

"I'll be out in a couple days. I don't think I need *that*."

"Up to you, my friend."

The tiny kit containing holy oils, holy water, and candles—which he keeps in his glove compartment and had brought into the hospital in anticipation—remained in Father Greer's suit pocket.

As we left the room, Father Greer shook his head. "It's so hard." We walked farther down the corridor, and he took the stole from around his neck and folded it. "Just to accept our weakness. So hard to accept God's power. We all fight it."

"The illness, the illness; why does something like that have to happen just to make you wake up to who you really are?"

We sat talking in the living room of his suite at the rectory one evening. Although I had tried a few times before to have Father Greer reflect on his life, his work, and his illness, he had deflected my questions, answering with sweeping generalities. He was a priest, an average one at best; this was what he did. He had had good medical care; he was hoping for the best. But that evening, after a day that had included an appointment with Dr. Desforges at New England Medical Center as well as hospital rounds in Natick, he was somehow different. I would not say anything had changed so dramatically in his life that he wanted finally to unburden himself. It seemed, rather, that he had simply become ready to put into words what he had been thinking about for some time.

"I was told I might die. I was told that even if the medication worked, I would never be cancer-free; it would only be in remission. I thought I was totally in control of my life: in great shape, a jogger, swimmer, golfer, only a few pounds heavier than when I was ordained. Death was for the other fellow; those were the people I was helping, and let's emphasize the 'I.' There is a kind of professional compassion, and I was good at it, but I could never really feel what it was to be on the receiving end, the needy side. I was, in a sense, taught to do it unemotionally, and I could do that, mechanically go through the motions. I hate to admit that, but sometimes it's the best you have; it's a job and you have to do it however you happen to be feeling at the time. Often you are emotionally drained. I think I was sometimes cold with people in the hospitals; I never physically touched them. Now I don't find that so hard. Like with poor Jenny going off to the operating room.

"We priests talk humility, but a kind of arrogance is closer to the truth. Suddenly I knew what it was like to be in a hospital bed, sure the doctors weren't telling you everything. Suddenly I realized Joe Greer wasn't in charge anymore. I had already faced the fact that the world wasn't black and white and that Father didn't have all the answers. But the illness made me aware of the fragility, the impermanence of all of us. It made me appreciate the Sacrament of the Sick and what a beautiful stepping-stone it is—either back to healthy life or on to the next life. Having received it myself, I can understand its power. That's why I want it for others and want them to understand what it is. It's not the closing of the coffin; it's that stepping-stone. After a year and a half on the medication, they told me there is no trace of my disease; I'm clear. But it's not really gone, and I know that. Impermanence, all over again.

"Facing death, you try to make all sorts of bargains with God. About what you'll do if He just lets you get better. For me, it's not an issue of going to heaven or to hell. I've thought about that over the years, and I've come to the conclusion that He sent His Son to save us. He's not going to let anyone slip between the cracks.

"So I stopped trying to bargain with God. I don't try to be any different, or look more holy than I ever was—which is not all that holy, believe me. If I have anything, it comes out in my humanity and in my work, not out of my mouth.

"I just said to God I'd try to be the best priest I could if I had any time left." He hesitated, as if he had finished.

"He gave me that time."

7

This deception of mine has been quite successful, and I notice how readily people believe me as soon as I say that I feel quite well.

Father Greer claims to be, and is, an intensely private man. He has legions of admirers, but few close friends. Some of the latter are priests—Father James Canniff of St. Mary's, Charlestown, is one, as well as his partners-in-ownership of a modest ski chalet in New Hampshire, Fathers Thomas Fleming of St. Brigid's, South Boston, and William O'Connor of St. Paul's, Wellesley. There are a handful of couples who have crossed over the undrawn but manifest line between clergy and laity and are now friends—former parishioners like the Hajjars and the Colas, and a few in the current parish, like the Garveys and the Barrys. Janet Hamilton, the church secretary, is far more than an employee. And Father Greer lives in daily contact with two younger priests in what is supposed to be a small clerical community.

It is a measure of his level of privacy that from the moment he was diagnosed with multiple myeloma and began treatment, except for the times he required emergency transportation when he was physically unable to drive, he asked none of the people who might be considered closest to him to accompany him into the hospital for any of the many tests and clinic visits a patient with such a disease must endure.

After his initial hospitalizations in both Natick and Boston, and then during the many months of frequent examinations and treatments at the clinic, he was willing to answer direct questions about his illness and treatment, but usually in the most general of terms and in a manner that did not invite further inquiry. And so even those who lived with him could only speculate about his well-being.

Father Mullaney: "There is that dark Irish side to Joe; his face seems frozen; he won't say much about it. He was so obviously going through a heavy, heavy depression after he found out what he had, but you don't know what to do about it. It really can't be addressed. That is the last thing you would do: 'Not feeling too chipper, Joe; want to talk about it?' We had all seen the dark side of him before, when things were going badly in the parish, but he couldn't seem to shake this one; it was 'Father Gloom-and-Doom' all the time, and we felt so inadequate to do anything about it."

Father Rossi: "When he came back from the first stay in the hospital, after he had the diagnosis, he wouldn't say much about how he felt, but he started talking more and more about this priest with leukemia, or that one who died so unexpectedly. It was all very indirect. I think it was the best he could do to express the real feelings that were going on inside him. I think because we all respect and admire him so much, there isn't anything we wouldn't do for him to help him through these days. But there just doesn't seem to be any good way to do it, except to try not to lapse into morbidness. I'm not saying that we want to run around with a silly grin on our faces, but we try to keep conversation on the most pleasant things we can."

Janet Hamilton: "There seemed to be a heaviness about him. You would just catch him with a certain look on his face that was so grim. But if you asked how he was feeling, he would shrug it off and get right on with business. He has never been a person to talk about himself—he always switches the conversation around to the other person—and damned if this was going to change him."

And so no one had a clear picture of exactly what he was going through. No one had met his doctors, no one had even gone inside the waiting room of the clinic he regularly visited.

Customarily, to avoid the morning rush hour traffic, Father Greer would drive into Charlestown on the evening before an appointment, park his car in the St. Mary's lot, and spend the night in the rectory before Father Canniff dropped him off at the medical center the next morning. When he was through, he would call Father Canniff to be taken back to his car and then would drive back to Natick.

I do not want to imply that Father Greer had come to trust me in some unique way that allowed me, after about half a year of knowing him, to be his companion on his clinic visits. That was not my understanding. I think it was simply because I asked him if I might go along, something those who knew him much better than I did would never have presumed to do.

The hematology/oncology clinic waiting room at the New England Medical Center, which had become so familiar to him during the past year and a half, is a light, airy area on the third floor of the Biewend Building. Its walls, painted an appealing shade of dusty rose, are enhanced with prints from the Boston Museum of Art. At about nine-thirty on the appointed days—usually Tuesdays— "Greer, Fr. Joseph" would present his battered plastic identification card at the desk and receive a sheaf of medical forms and multi-colored lab slips. He would wait, usually no more than fifteen minutes, to have three to five vials of blood drawn by a technician wearing rubber gloves (since the advent of AIDS) and then take a seat to await the next calling of his name, meaning that his physician was ready to see him.

On a midautumn morning, one that was uncharacteristically cold and blustery, Father Greer was wearing a white windbreaker, bright yellow trousers, and a pair of topsiders. He never wore clerical clothing to the medical center. He had brought along the Weakland book on the post–Vatican II church. He looked up only occasionally and seemed intent on reading, but he rarely turned the page. Patients shuffled across the carpeted floor or were pushed in wheelchairs, studies in slow motion. In contrast, staff members moved through the room rapidly, purposefully. Across from Father Greer was a young boy whose peach fuzz was still not thick enough to hide the huge scar over his left ear. Two seats to his left, a teenage girl sat wearing a baseball hat to cover her head, bald from radiation or chemotherapy or both. On the other side of the room were two older men accompanied by their wives. Father Greer had seen these couples here for months; he waved and said hello.

In general, there was little conversation between patients and family members. What sounds there were came from the staff: their own conversations and the occasional call of a patient's name.

Though Father Greer, following his third or fourth visit, had dubbed the waiting room in Biewend 3 the "depression room," this morning a smile came to his face. There were fewer people in the room than usual. "Must have all gone to Fatima to be cured," he commented.

He was summoned by Dr. John Erban, a resident fellow who functions as Father Greer's primary physician under the direction of Dr. Desforges. Dr. Erban is a short, always mildly fatigued but perennially smiling young man whose tousled brown hair seems constantly in need of a trim. From the first meeting he insisted on being called "Jack."

"Keeping up with the swimming, are you, Father Greer?" he asked as the patient took off his shirt.

"Maybe twice a week, when I can get away from the buzz saw."

"Good, good. Gone back to jogging?"

"Oh, no. I think I'll wait awhile for that one."

"Whatever. We see a profound change in people who exercise, so keep it up." As he talked, Dr. Erban took Father Greer's blood pressure and then with his hands checked Father Greer's neck glands and his torso, pressing in repeatedly at the location of his liver and spleen. He listened to his heartbeat with a stethoscope and spent considerable time passing it over the front and back of Father Greer's lungs.

"Good, good, nice and clear. The appetite? Your weight?"

"Sorry to say it's got a stranglehold on 195. I was 169 out of the sem, 175 at my twenty-fifth reunion, and, whang, it popped up to 195 and won't budge."

"We can thank the prednisone for that. Great drug, but it gives you a voracious appetite and then your body gets used to extra weight. But we're through with the prednisone now. That weight should come off within a year. Any other problems?"

"Well, I'm tired all the time, don't have the old zip. Had a sore throat and can't seem to shake it. And the pain back here," he said, placing his hand on the back of his waist on the right side.

"Does the Motrin control it?"

"When I take it, I guess, but I don't like to get dependent on painkillers."

"Don't be afraid to use it, Father Greer; it will help to make you comfortable. The last X rays we took of your back didn't show any porosity due to the myeloma, so we think it's a rheumatism that's the cause."

Dr. Desforges knocked, then entered the room. She is a tall, trim, striking woman of sixty-seven with gray hair that she wears in a youthful pageboy, the ends saucily curled. In her long white hospital coat she is thoroughly professional, but also—because of an infectious, embracing smile—quite motherly. "And how is our Father Greer today?" she asked cheerily.

"Blood pressure of an athlete; 110 over 56," said Dr. Erban.

"Some athlete," Father Greer said with a weary smile. "I looked at my jogging suit in the closet and put an RIP on it."

"But you're still swimming and walking; you look in wonderful condition," said Dr. Desforges.

"Father Greer is complaining of fatigue and that backache," Dr. Erban said. "But the lungs are nice and clear."

"As you know, Father Greer, the myeloma is the overgrowth of one kind of cell in the marrow and sometimes that weakens the bones, but our best guess is that you have a little persistent rheumatism in there," said Dr. Desforges. "The overgrowth also causes anemia, and that causes a person to feel run-down more quickly. Also, your ability to fight infection is reduced, so we have to keep an eye on that. But I just checked the blood we drew today and your counts are fine, excellent in fact; better than last time. The myeloma is in remission."

"Remission." Father Greer's voice was flat.

"And that's where we want it to stay. So if you feel any different or old symptoms return, let us know immediately. Don't hesitate to call, because if it comes back, we want to begin to treat it again as soon as possible. And the rest of your life? Are you getting your days off, getting up to New Hampshire?"

"I had three days planned last week to get away. Never made it. Out to the links to beat the ball around, that's the best I could do."

"Please try to cut back. I sent a letter off to the archdiocese that explains your condition."

"Oh, they'll read it, all right, and then what? There isn't exactly a bullpen full of relief pitchers out there ready to come in."

"Really, Father Greer, when you are overtired, the disease is more likely to take advantage of that."

"Oh, I take a snooze in the afternoon once in a while; I'm doing better."

"An event in your life like this tells you you can't do the things you did when you were thirty or forty. Now you can do what you please. You can live more sensibly."

Father Greer smiled broadly. "Tell my desk calendar that. And the contractors and the cemetery workers and the people who want ten Masses every Sunday morning, at convenient times, of course."

"But you must see to your own needs; take care of yourself. After all—"

"You're being very pastoral, doctor. I thought that was my line of work."

Dr. Desforges blinked behind her thick glasses; there was a flush of red to her high cheekbones. "We want you to do well, Father Greer; that's the important thing. There is this sword hanging over your head, we all know that. I just want you to be in the best possible condition."

"I just never thought of it," he said, smiling, "as a nine-to-five job."

8

Salt stings an open wound, but saves you from gangrene.

Father Greer's three-room suite on the second floor of St. Patrick's rectory, decorated at his direction in a restful shade approaching Wedgwood blue, is a large, handsome bachelor apartment. His living room has a comfortable sofa, two easy chairs, and a lounger, which sits across the room from a television and stereo console. Between the living room and his office is a narrow room that holds a small bar with refrigerator beneath. There are always potato chips and peanuts, plenty of clean glasses, soft drinks, and beer, as well as a stock of bourbon and sweet vermouth—and the cherries—that go to make Manhattans, Father Greer's drink of choice. Off the living room is a bathroom, with a second one adjoining his bedroom at the opposite end of his office.

Two large plants dominate the living room. One of them contains a tiny gray stuffed raccoon that peers out partly hidden between perfect plastic branches. In a corner stands a small library of Father Greer's books, combining such seminary stalwarts as Dom Marmion and more currently popular authors like Hans Küng. A few mementoes of his years in the priesthood decorate the walls. One is a needlepoint map of the Boston area showing the location and the year he arrived at each of the six churches he served before coming to St. Patrick's: St. Joseph's in Quincy, 1958; St. Catherine's, Norwood, 1964; St. James, Boston, 1968; St. Anthony's, Cohasset, 1969; St. Mark's, Dorchester, 1970; and St. Joseph's, Hyde Park,

1977. It is inscribed "Lord, Make Me an Instrument of Your Peace" and was given to the priest on the occasion of the twenty-fifth anniversary of his ordination by St. Joseph's parishioners. There are a few citations on the walls, among them one acknowledging Father Greer's attendance at a four-month clergy education program in Menlo Park, California. There is a plaque from the Boston City Council "in honor of outstanding service to Hyde Park and his work for racial harmony." It rests on the floor, Father Greer not having found a place to hang it. There are a few photographs: his 1958 St. John's Seminary class picture is on the wall; on a table is a photo taken at the twenty-fifth reunion of that same class, now reduced by a third, standing around Cardinal Medeiros.

While it is a most inviting and spacious place, it is also the location of two Touch-Tone telephones—one on his desk, one beside the lounge chair—each with a built-in intercom and three extensions. Beyond the doors that open out from his office and the living room onto a carpeted hallway is a flight of stairs leading to the rectory's busy first floor.

Shortly after he arrived at St. Patrick's, Father Greer insisted that the pastor's quarters be refurbished, redecorated, and expanded. He found them claustrophobic and dingy. And while he is pleased with his present lodging, he, like the vast majority of parish priests, does not call his part of the rectory "home." Clergy of more recent vintage tend to spend days off at their parents', men of Father Greer's generation at a privately owned cottage or home.

Father Greer's home away from what is not quite home is a two-and-a-half-hour drive almost directly north of Boston. After Mass on a Wednesday morning, on the first of his scheduled two days off, we left Natick and drove toward Father Greer's cottage in Franconia, New Hampshire. I was interested to see him outside the rectory and in a relaxed setting, but I also wanted to be able to sit down and talk at length with him and not be interrupted by the appointments that make up his day and the calls that perforate his schedule at will.

We drove up Interstate 93 with WJIB playing on the radio for most of the trip. Father Greer proved to be a knowledgeable tour guide, making comments on everything from the spate of newly constructed buildings along Route 128—spawned first by the Boston area's high-technology boom but currently in a slight downturn, as the many FOR LEASE signs testify—to the Old Man of the Mountain in New Hampshire, a huge natural outcropping of rock in the configuration of a human profile that constitutes a landmark and a local tourist attraction. In the summer, Father Greer is an avid golfer who usually hits in the high eighties; in the winter, a rather accomplished skier. It was the desire to have a getaway that would allow them to indulge their passion for skiing that led the three priests to this location in the White Mountains, close to Cannon Mountain Ski Area. And being priests, who take their days off during the week as Saturdays and Sundays are far too jammed with Masses, weddings, and baptisms, they can indulge their passion without having to deal with the crowds that hamper the weekend skier.

As we drove I wondered if the Father Greer I had gotten to know better and better during our time together would change when we began to speak at length about his church, his priesthood, and what sustains him, topics that, despite our efforts, had proven difficult to tackle during the hectic days in Natick and, once the evening and the warming effects of a couple of Manhattans had enfolded us, impossible. He had never failed to answer my questions, but those questions had been specific and limited, to help me understand something he had done.

I noted Father Greer's candor, and I speculated as to whether or not it would be sustained. Such openness was a quality I had not found in great abundance in the dozens of priests—friends, classmates, and acquaintances—I had met through him. Often their answers to my occasional questions had been general, clerically distant, and unforthcoming, sometimes obscured by humor but sometimes defensive, as if they were editing their remarks as they spoke.

We turned off at Route 18 in Franconia, wound through a development called Lafayette Acres, and turned into a driveway at the sign listing "Fleming, O'Connor, Greer."

"Very appropriate," said Father Greer as we pulled in. "F-O-G. Fog."

The three priests are owners of a simple but comfortable three-bedroom batten-board chalet done predominantly in the beiges and browns that recall St. Patrick's third-floor common room. Many of the pieces of furniture are parishioners' castoffs or family hand-me-downs (heirlooms would be a dishonest assessment, Father Greer insisted), such as the walnut-veneer breakfront and table that once sat in his parents' dining room. Each morning he is here, Father Greer says Mass at this table, using recycled shrimp cocktail jars for cruets and a host kept fresh through damp weather and dry in a polyethylene bag in the refrigerator. Two squat candles and a vase of plastic flowers complete the makeshift altar.

I mentioned that the table must have sentimental value for him as it had seen so many Greer family meals. "Yes, it's seen a lot," he said, "and maybe, in its latest incarnation, a tear or two from all the priests who sat around it."

We took a long walk after lunch, and in the periods of extended silence, with which we both had grown comfortable, I asked myself: What do I know of this man so far?

On one hand, he is a loyal priest of whom his pope and archbishop can justly be proud, a company man not reluctant to proclaim the absoluteness of church teaching. And yet I had found that after shooting off a moralistic salvo or judgment, he often hastens to apply the balm of exculpation.

He is a man who has pushed past the boundaries of his priesthood, tasted pleasures forbidden him, violated his vows, witnessed the raw exercise of church power, seen his best friends leave, and yet has remained a priest—and a certain kind of priest. He is neither an updated version of a benevolent Bing Crosby in *Going My Way* nor a throwback who pretends—as some priests are pleased to do with a doctrinal pope in command—that the past twenty-five years never happened. Nor is he an efficient clerical CEO who avoids the vagaries of the spiritual life while seeing to the administration of a large parish. I often saw him angry with his church and his superiors, but never embittered. He is forbearing and philosophical about the human failings of this divinely inspired institution, the church, but never acquiescent.

It was midafternoon when we finally sat down to talk. I began by asking him how he and his church had changed since his ordination.

"Sometimes this is a church that expects too much of her people," he said as he gazed out at a barren Cannon Mountain. He was wearing trousers, shirt, and sweater in graduated shades of mustard and yellow along with a pair of topsiders. "I never thought I'd live to see the day I'd say that, because at one time it was so easy to judge; I was right and they were wrong. I was willing to be measured by the toughest standards, and I imposed them on other people. Then came the sixties and seventies and I found I was just as weak as the weakest of them. Pathetically weak. Now I'm not so quick to judge. I don't want to be judged that harshly myself. Maybe I'm a little late as I'm rounding third and heading for home, but I hope I'm learning that the true sign of the church is forgiveness, not to make the wounds deeper.

"I look at some of my closest friends, ex-priests, good, decent men. Present church policy makes it difficult to release them from their vows, and if they are not laicized they can't be married in the eyes of the church nor can they function in the church or receive the Eucharist. They are in limbo, unforgiven sinners. And when they are laicized, they aren't allowed to function as priests anymore, as the majority of them want to do. I feel their enormous pain as they live as outcasts. I see people who've had a bad marriage because partners didn't live up to their side of the bargain; they're supposed to suffer with that for the rest of their lives? Or marry again and not be able to receive Our Lord in the Eucharist? I know of a parishioner who faithfully attended daily Mass for thirty years, yet who couldn't officially take Communion because of a terrible and short first marriage the bureaucracy couldn't find the inclination to annul.

"A fellow ordained around my time is the first Boston diocesan priest with AIDS. Compassion? The first reaction was to ask him to leave his parish. Where's Our Lord's love in that? For a man who served all those years? Sometimes the church is the older brother in the story of the Prodigal Son: 'You never gave me a break; you did what you wanted to do, and now you're going to pay for it.' God is kinder to man than man is to himself.

"I think that's why many parish priests today don't pay a whole lot of attention to what's coming down from Rome or from the chancery. You can't take all of it seriously and keep your sanity. I know priests who haven't opened chancery mail in two months. Personally, I save mine for after supper when I can have a healthy glass of Scotch in my mitt. There's a constant tug-o'-war that goes on, where the chancery demands reports exactly on time, tells you to send money for your kids who go to other parochial schools, wants more subscriptions for the revamped diocesan newspaper, *The Pilot*—which, incidentally, is, shall we say, 'closely scrutinized by church authorities.' You're supposed to start married and separated clubs, volunteer for seminarian confessions; there's no end to the demands. We hear so much talk about the diocese as a community, but if you want to have a community, the leader has to earn his authority as the pastor must earn his. I think Archbishop Bernadin in Chicago and Bishop Hunthausen out in Seattle—although I don't agree with all their views—have merited their priests' respect. It doesn't work by edict any more. Those two fellows really try to achieve collegiality, meanwhile living the spirit of Vatican II. They are open, not afraid of change.

"I've had direct experience with our present archbishop, Cardinal Law, and with his predecessor, Cardinal Medeiros, so I know first-hand why priests get worn down by the system and why all the so-called consultations and synods usually don't add up to much. Take the recent Vatican synod on the laity. Meetings all over the archdiocese; position papers drawn up. Planeloads of people go to Rome. The result? Nothing to brag about.

"When I was on the Priests' Council in the nineteen-seventies, we all believed we were going to reform the system from within. Cardinal Medeiros—a holy man to be sure, yet once that miter goes up on top of a man's head funny things happen—asked me to hold a special election among the priests to choose a clergy personnel director. There was a lot of dissatisfaction with who was being sent where and why. Then the cardinal informed me, regardless of the outcome, he would keep his man in the office. I protested in no uncertain terms about the charade he was putting me through, but he said 'Do it.' Under obedience, I held the election. And his man won anyhow, but something was lost in that process. Later he asked for a survey on the personnel department and its workings and I thought, 'Aha, we'll get it out *this* way!' I had a questionnaire drawn up by a top sociologist, sent it out to all the priests in the archdiocese, and proudly presented it to the cardinal. He didn't like what it told him—that priests were no longer willing to be moved around as he and his inner circle saw fit—and he refused to have it published. The personnel situation appears to be better today, though. Priests may be overworked, but they at least have a say in *where* they're overworked.

"In the early days at St. Patrick's, when we were trying to get this place moving again, I spent an entire year in a parish renewal, which was capped off by five consecutive nights where an average of seven hundred people turned out, because they cared so much about their parish. The following Sunday, every priest at every Mass was to preach about the renewal. It so happened Cardinal Law had sent out a tape on abortion he wanted played that Sunday and when I didn't, one of my kindly parishioners turned me in. The cardinal was on the phone asking me, 'Is there a reason for this?' I told him about the renewal, the state of the parish, and that I'd made a pastoral judgment. He wasn't very impressed with my judgment and told me it was more important to have continuity—that my decision showed me and my parish to be out of step with him. I tried to explain further, but he just got angry. Now, this is the same man who, during my illness, was a frequent visitor and often called to see how I was doing. He was wonderful. He is very pastoral toward his priests. I just can't understand it, so I just don't even try anymore. But to any criticism I might make I would immediately add that these men have brutal schedules, enormous pressures on them— and, often, lonely lives. I just visited a priest about my age who is now a bishop, and he lives alone in a big place, no housekeeper, and is having a hard time being accepted by his priests because he's an Easterner, an outsider to them. He asked me to concelebrate Mass, then to have breakfast, then to do other things with him. I could see he was starved for companionship. It made me very sad for him. We priests have each other—for better or worse, there is the clerical club. But when you get up there as a bishop, there's not so many of you around.

"I'll never forget how happy Boston priests were when Law was named our archbishop. Here was a man with the stature, the look the archdiocese rated. Poor Cardinal Medeiros was never accepted, a Portuguese, that kind of outsider. Believe me, a lot of us felt guilty when we laid that man in his grave. Priests bucked his rulings, like admitting white kids to their parochial schools who were doing nothing but looking for a way to escape going to an integrated public school. But Medeiros at least seemed open. With Law, you wonder if he doesn't have his agenda set, regardless of what might be needed or wanted. The chancery sends out a form every couple of years for us to recommend the names of possible new bishops. I really don't pay much attention to this process.

"Priests are bucking their superiors, and the laity, a much higher quality laity than we ever had before, aren't listening to the church anymore. You might trace a lot of it back to Pope Paul VI's encyclical *Humanae Vitae*, which forbade the use of birth control at a time when sixty expert consultants hired by the Vatican were in favor of it and the practice was widespread anyhow. When you look at Vatican proclamations, you have to consider two elements: one is *Ecclesia docens*, the church teaching, and the second is the *sensus fidelium*, the response of the faithful, or, in effect, the church listening. If the teaching has no listeners, that says something about the validity of what is being said; the listeners are saying something to the teachers. The *sensus fidelium* was that *Humanae Vitae* was off base, and they basically ignored it. But sadly, some people left the church because of it. I'm not for some watered-down, convenient religious faith. The salt without savor. But this is not the world it was when Joe Greer first put on the biretta up there at St. John's.

"I can still remember when *Humanae Vitae* was issued. I was giving pre-Cana marriage conferences in Boston, and naturally these young couples were asking me about it. I defended it. I was scraping the bottom of the theological barrel to come up with arguments, but I did it. I suppose I was double-talking them. You learn; you grow up; you think. Now if someone asks about birth control, I give chapter and verse on *Humanae Vitae* and then listen for extenuating circumstances. I usually hear some." He smiled.

"This thing called celibacy, when will it go? I wish it had gone yesterday. Not for old Father Greer—although I have to admit I'd give marriage a thought; the old dog knows a nice ankle and a pretty face when he sees one and whether hemlines are going up or down— but for the many fine young men it keeps from becoming priests. I don't think you're a better priest because you're celibate. Yes, it is a beautiful gift to present to God and it stands as a sign of your commitment to serve all people while you yourself do not have a wife and family. But you don't find too many priests my age standing up and proclaiming celibacy must be maintained. We older priests know that the quality and quantity of men aspiring to the priesthood would be greatly improved and that this tendency toward the feminizing of the clergy would be checked. I find it very hard to be convincing about celibacy when a young man comes to me, talking about the priesthood. I just can't lie to him that it is all that important anymore.

"My own violations of the vow took me to some of the lowest points in my life, but—hindsight, you are so wise!—they had a profound effect on my priesthood. I had never understood before how people could fall and then fall again. But I learned over a half-dozen years of falling and falling again myself. I learned not to love people because they are perfect, and I learned that as God forgave me, the least I could do was reciprocate with the people I serve. I learned from my own mistakes that people don't really *want* to sin. I learned how wretched you can feel about yourself, how low you can be, how down.

"But I never hesitated to see a priest and go to confession after I'd sinned; I needed the sign of God's love. And through it all—this is strange to say—I knew myself. I knew I was born to be a priest of God. And I would die one. In my falling I was raised up to a new life. It was like a baptism to me.

"I guess I know as sure as I know anything, I was called to the priesthood, to be in the world but not of it, to serve. A great ideal, but it's the height of peace and joy. It plainly makes you feel good. But it didn't take long for me to realize that it could extract an enormous toll. You were crying when I buried that baby, and you asked how I could go through that without showing my emotions. I see so much grief every week that, although each case is unique, there is a commonness about them. I have to convince myself of that because my emotions couldn't stand the strain if I got involved each time. I remember my first funeral, at St. Joseph's in Quincy. I came back to the rectory with tears in my eyes, and the pastor, Monsignor Allston, a great man, took me aside and said, 'Father, if you want to survive, stop that right now! Toward the dead, you must be dead to yourself.'

"You learn to keep a check on your emotions, but the harder

part of the priesthood to deal with is a certain kind of deception that is the downfall of most of us: we have the ideal and actually think *we* can will ourselves to live up to it. That if we work harder and longer we'll be better and better priests. It took having the cancer, being so sick, for me to finally acknowledge the source of strength and health. I used to be a bit of a workaholic. The Lord must really have been smiling down on Joe Greer flailing around down here! I don't know if I'm any better a priest now, but I'm not so worried about it. I can go about it gently. I can be a pastor and roll with the punches, know that I'm going to lose most of the battles, but that it's not up to me anymore. The illness. It taught me. Not about death, but about dependence.

"I'll be at St. Patrick's for a while, then maybe an assistant someplace, but I see myself functioning as a priest right into my retirement. I love this little cabin; I love being up here away from all the problems, and God knows I love to ski, but I love even more doing what I do.

"Someday, when I'm retired, I'll want to serve a small parish three or four days a week. With the shortage, I'm sure there'll be a spot for the toddling old Joe Greer."

9

"It's for your own good. When you've lived longer, you will understand, but you'll have to live . . ."

"Have to live!" I answered without thinking. "An awful thought, isn't it?"

What continually struck me as I spent time with Father Greer was that this parish priest was both a terribly overworked man in an understaffed church and a man afflicted by a disease for which there was no cure, but that neither the Catholic Church in Boston nor Joseph Greer in person appeared to be in any imminent danger of collapse. For all the troubles, each seemed to be functioning at a high level of service, efficiency, and grace. As for St. Patrick's— and, I assumed, parishes throughout the Boston Archdiocese and across America—Masses were being said, spiritual and temporal needs met, buildings kept in some state of repair; Catholics were brought into the church in baptism, laid to rest in burial, joined in Holy Matrimony. Confessions were heard, bingo played. Using as my template the Beatitudes that Father Greer often called the basis of his ministry, the hungry were fed, the homeless sheltered, and prisoners, if not visited, were certainly welcomed and helped upon their release.

As for this man with a fatal disease, I saw a priest with not a sword over his head but a goal before him—to revitalize as many members of a large congregation as he could reach and to refurbish a parish's physical plant.

And so, to better understand this paradox, I made a plan: to revisit places Father Greer and I had gone together to pay calls—alone—on those people who might put it in perspective for me. After all, the Catholic Church in America had experienced a serious drop in the number of priests. Why was it that a parish within that monolith could function so well with such a limited staff? And how was it that this man, Father Greer, not one to be overly or stupidly optimistic about anything in life, could go on with such imperturbable aplomb?

Before returning to the sprawling archdiocesan complex on Commonwealth Avenue and the office of Father James McCarthy, the director of clergy personnel, I thought it wise to do some basic research on Catholics and the priests who serve them.

According to *The Official Catholic Directory*, there are today in the United States some 19,500 parishes in 185 dioceses. While St. Patrick's ranks among the larger parishes, the average Catholic parish consists of some 2,300 people. This number seems even more substantial when compared to Protestant churches, 50 to 75 percent of which have no more than five hundred members. In the Episcopal Church, there are 245 laypersons per full-time priest, in the American Lutheran Church, 372. In the Catholic Church, the figure is 912. And so, while the pace of Father Greer's days and nights is certainly of his own making—he has always been a driven man to whom idleness was more tiresome than work—it is also a necessity. He has a lot of people to look after.

There are other key differences between the Catholic and Protestant clergy: the Catholic priest usually resides next door to his church and, as a celibate, has no family to tend or shield him from whoever may call on him or whatever unpleasant tasks he may have to perform. His parish is his bride and his life, and within that parish the parishioners' assumption is that there is a priest available twenty-four hours a day.

The Second Vatican Council fostered a shift away from strict authoritarian rule by priests and passive attendance at religious rituals by laity so that a "people of God," in the spirit of the early church, might again be assembled. This, indeed, has happened at St. Patrick's and, to some degree, at most Catholic churches. Catholic laypeople have a considerable say in their church today, and significant liturgical and ministerial roles as Eucharistic ministers, lectors, counselors, educators, and administrators.

But the shift is incomplete. The priest is still the only one who can say Mass and perform certain sacraments and, as surveys have consistently shown, it is to him that Catholics still turn in their moments of grief, celebration, and need. (There is a growing but not yet widespread trend to hire professional administrators to oversee a parish's business affairs, but this practice, besides being expensive for churches to underwrite, is felt as an affront by the men of Father Greer's generation.)

In the aftermath of the Second Vatican Council, when attendance at Mass dropped precipitously, it might have been assumed that the numbers of Catholics had gone down. Just the opposite is true. The number of Catholics has actually risen dramatically: the Gallup poll has found that there are 64 million, up 17 million—some 30 percent—in the last twenty years. This increase is due to an influx of Catholic immigrants, primarily from Central America, the Caribbean, and Mexico, plus ordinary growth in U.S. Catholic families. And while the modern-day Catholic may not be the churchgoer he or she would have been twenty years ago, when a child is born, a marriage is to take place, or someone is to be buried, the nominal Catholic returns for the ritual. This is why Father Greer baptizes, marries, and buries scores of people he does not know.

At least officially, the decline in the number of priests does not *seem* to be as dramatic. According to *The Official Catholic Directory*, in 1967 there were 59,892 priests; in 1989 there were 52,948, a drop of 11 percent. In contrast, independent surveys have indicated that, conservatively, between 12 and 17 percent of American clergy ceased functioning as priests during that period. Of course, the figures don't jibe, and when I arrived I asked Father McCarthy about that.

"Ah, statistics," he said in a voice that indicated he would willingly be a true believer in numbers if, indeed, numbers equaled priests. "I can't go down those fifty-odd-thousand names and tell you how many are retired or ill or inactive or have simply left the priesthood without doing it formally. All I can point to with any surety are the figures here in Boston. In 1971, which incidentally was the first year for which we have any solid numbers—before that there were so many priests to go around, nobody needed to count them—we had 1,317 active diocesan priests. Today, we have 945. And there are 407 parishes in the archdiocese, containing from twenty-five thousand people to no more than five hundred.

"We could perhaps respond better to the current crisis, but the church unfortunately is still in the 'all things to all people' phase, something we could handle when we had a surfeit of priests. It is a noble ideal, a keystone of our diocesan priesthood—Father was supposed to say 'yes' to every request. Vatican II brought about a basic, time-consuming process of reeducation both for the laity— who are growing—and the priests—who are shrinking. What did the old priest have to know about Liturgy? He said his standard Mass, that was it. Counseling? He recited dogma. Long-range planning, good administrative techniques, accountability? He collected money and spent it. Cash and carry. Social concerns, social awareness? In a parish ninety-nine and forty-four hundredths percent pure Irish or Italian, what did you need to know about that stuff?

"I have openings in churches right now that can't be filled. The diocese has tried to cut back the number of priests in each parish on some rational basis—we use a 'sacramental index,' where we add up the number of baptisms, deaths, and marriages—marriages times two, and if the number is below 125 and the church's population below 3,125 we assign one priest; below 300 on the index and less than 7,500 people, two priests; 499 and 12,500, three priests; 500 and above and more than 12,501 people, four priests. At best, it is arbitrary.

"Every priest out there is stretched, and—and—" he seemed bemused at the thought coming up "—it's so hard to find men out there with a combination of the needed skills, men like your priest, Joe Greer. I wouldn't mind thirty or forty Joe Greers right now. I'd have them in a parish by the weekend.

"All right, 975 priests, 407 parishes. We're getting by, but don't forget, Joe Greer's time was the golden era, record numbers of priests. What happens when they reach their sixties and seventies and begin to retire in substantial numbers? We are here," Father McCarthy said, his hand at eye level, "and, because we experience a net loss every year, with thirty to thirty-five priests either retiring, dying, leaving, or becoming incapacitated and only ten to fifteen new men being ordained, our numbers go down." His hand glided gently to a plane even with his chin. "We float along, losing a little altitude." The hand was now on a slightly lower plane, at the top of his crisp Roman collar. "In ten years, maybe twelve . . ." His hand fell, as if struck, to the top of his desk.

"I think an appropriate word would be precipitous."

I was interested in other opinions on the state of the clergy and went to see two men who could "bracket" Father McCarthy's assessment. Each is uniquely qualified to address the issue: one a member of the Boston hierarchy, a man organizationally above Father McCarthy; the other beneath him, outside the ranks of parish priests, but skilled in analyzing trends.

The Most Reverend Robert Banks is one of Boston's five auxiliary bishops, the archdiocesan vicar general, and the vicar for administration. On an organizational chart, he is directly below Bernard Cardinal Law. Bishop Banks is a handsome, grey-haired cleric who wears meticulously tailored suits and greets visitors to his uncluttered, spacious office with a warm smile and handshake. The office is in the main chancery building, located between the seminary, with the ever-smaller number of men in its pipeline, and the Tribunal Building, where Father McCarthy sits with lists of clergy openings he cannot fill.

"Yes, it is a problem, we all know that," Bishop Banks said in an even, controlled voice, "but to me, a small problem and not really alarming. History. We have to have some sense of history. This is an ancient and venerable institution which has seen many feasts and famines in two thousand years. It's necessary to keep some perspective on this and realize there will not be a *real* shortage for ten or fifteen years. And that to make foolish compromises just to boost the numbers is to deny God the opportunity to solve still another problem of this puny thing called man which he created. Fifteen years ago we had plenty of priests. Why not again, fifteen years from now?"

I summarized Bishop Banks's assessment for Father Michael Groden, the director of the Archdiocesan Planning Office for Urban Affairs, and asked for his opinion. He is a Harvard-trained public policy analyst whose office is in downtown Boston, near the Faneuil Hall Market.

Father Groden seemed unable to sit down during our conversation. We began well past the appointment time, and therefore he would be late for his next commitment, which was on the other side of the city. Father Groden's office was virtually wallpapered with tiny yellow notes to himself reminding him of tasks undone, phone calls not returned.

"Change is painful for an old, large institution, and if you don't have the imagination, guts, vision, and intelligence, you postpone it with 'Yes, this is a bit of a problem, and we'll address it later.' Boston is not alone in this matter, the church all across the country is doing the same thing. But let's be clear about this: it is not a matter of combining a couple of parishes or appointing a lay administrator [two examples Bishop Banks had given of archdiocesan experimentation], but of fundamental change. A large percentage of the students at Harvard Divinity School are Catholic. The men among them will not be priests, but obviously they are interested in religion. These are the people who very probably would have been in the seminary years ago. Now what is the archdiocese doing about them? Nothing," he uttered, finally sitting down, seemingly driven to exhaustion by the reality.

"There is an enormous reservoir of ex-priests, some seventeen thousand nationwide; a good number are right here in Boston. What about them? Nothing. The archdiocese never had to plan ahead, and they're not willing to do it now. Silence and inertia reign.

"And the real victim? That poor priest out in the parish. He doesn't feel appreciated by the hierarchy, a hierarchy which feels it can still pile more and more work on him. And when a priest comes back with a request for money or manpower, the answer is always no. We have a hundred and thirty-four one-priest parishes in Boston, something Cardinal Cushing absolutely forbade. He knew how hard it was for a priest to be living and functioning alone. But wait. In the years ahead, there'll be plenty more men alone out there."

My next stop was at St. John's Seminary and the office of the rector. "I'm quite pleased to be able to know our present-day seminarians so well—" the Reverend Thomas J. Daly began, chuckling, as we sat in his office within the huge edifice Cardinal Cushing had built with such optimism "—but I'd just as soon know more of them a little less." Father Daly is a cheery man with flushed cheeks, a veteran of thirty-four years in the Boston seminary system.

Last year he was appointed rector of St. John's. Currently, there are 118 Boston area men in formation: 50 in the final three years of theology and 68 in the first four years, known as philosophy, who take largely liberal arts courses. In Father Greer's day, there were between 400 and 450, some of them in the now defunct preparatory seminary in Jamaica Plain. In 1965, the peak year in America, there were 49,000 men in seminaries. Present enrollment is less than 9,000.

Outside his window, some Boston College coeds were availing themselves of an expanse of lawn to toss around a Frisbee in the warm afternoon air. Allowing women the use of seminary grounds is but the smallest of the changes here. "We are dealing with a different kind of candidate today," Father Daly said, "very, very different from Father Greer's day. This is the age of narcissism, a time when young men receive no peer group support. Yet they come to us. It is much more of an existential step off the plank, so we have to look at and train them accordingly. We realize they are more self-centered; we understand and are willing to support them if they, for instance, need therapy. In the old days, they would have been out the front door merely at the mention of it. We have an entire retreat devoted to celibacy. We want them prepared to deal with their sexuality, with living alone, which will happen to all of them, and probably soon. But above all, they must be professional. That's very important, we must have professional men."

If Father Daly seemed to be describing a sort of religious Foreign Legionnaire, the three seminarians selected for me to talk with (and I assumed because they were chosen they represented the seminary's best) gave me the impression that that is precisely the kind of mission for which they are readying themselves. Their curriculum seemed quite up to date, with much more psychology, less dogmatic theology and church history. It was certainly more liberal and far broader than it had been when Father Greer was at St. John's. Courses were offered in Ministry to the Divorced, Christian-Muslim Relations, and Protestant Ecclesiology—all of which would have been considered heretical in Father Greer's day—and the description of a Worship Practicum promised not mere orthodoxy, but help in developing a "celebration *style* for sacramental worship."

On the other hand, their outlook was reminiscent of 1950s staunchness. Surveys find many Catholic seminarians to be conservative, a word they bristled at, claiming to be "traditional" instead.

As I sat in an office with Kevin Devine, John Kearns, and Joseph Hennessey, three men close to ordination who had been selected by their coordinator of field education (interestingly enough a nun, Sister Mary O'Rourke), I heard the words that make Father Greer cringe. The soon-to-be priests want to "facilitate" and "empower"; they see themselves as "coordinators" who will "touch base" with the various lay staff and volunteers who will be doing much of the teaching, visiting, counseling, and distribution of Communion that was once the domain of the Catholic clergy. They will "take time to develop themselves within the ministerial framework." With such contemporary terminology on their lips, it was anomalous to hear them take such a hard line on celibacy, much harder than men of Father Greer's generation. They advocated continuing to bar ex-priests from presiding at Liturgies and were adamant about keeping women from the priesthood. They termed Vatican II a "gap" as well as a "bridge." This from young men who wanted to "bring more people into the circle." It is obviously a circle they will draw— or is it perhaps akin to a circle of pioneer wagons assembling for defense?

Looking at these bright, idealistic faces, which seemed to harden at the mention of issues currently at the center of church debate, I found myself confused. Perhaps they need to be steeled for the days ahead; it is a daunting future they face. But whoever the new Boston priest is, I found, he leaves St. John's *without* even a rudimentary knowledge of Latin—for centuries, the cornerstone of seminary education, regardless of its porosity—and *with* a propensity for the game of golf. During the 1960s and 1970s, the sport was as out of vogue as Hervé is today. Today, the men of St. John's, functionally illiterate in the ancient language of the church, are once again a company of golfers, captivated by the game that has provided companionship for Father Greer and his contemporaries as well as grist for clerical jokes.

To understand the church and priesthood, many points of view were needed; for the state of Father Greer's health, only one was really necessary.

Dr. Jane Desforges's small corner office is on the twelfth floor of the Tupper Building (named after the man who created Tupperware) at the New England Medical Center in Boston. As senior hematologist she has many administrative duties, but she spends a minimum amount of time in the office. She arrives for rounds before seven each morning, carries a full clinical load, does research, directs the fellows assigned to her, teaches in the Tufts Medical School, and lectures both in America and abroad.

"Father Greer came to us looking a bit pale, not all that sick, but now that I see how ruddy his complexion normally is, he really *was* looking poorly," she began. "His bone X rays showed less density in some spots but weren't all that striking. There was a mild anemia. In the blood we found a great buildup of monoclonal protein. And in the bone marrow there was an overgrowth of a clone of plasma cells, which is a sure indication of multiple myeloma.

"Multiple myeloma," she continued, giving a description she had undoubtedly rendered hundreds of times in her life, yet doing so without a trace of impatience or ennui, "is a cancer of the plasma cells found in the bone marrow, which normally produces antibodies for the immune system. These antibodies are what the body uses to fight infections, to attack the bacteria, the viruses to which all of us are constantly exposed.

"The body has great symmetry. The marrow is constantly producing a variety of cells, and in each cell there is DNA, which contains the program, if you will, that determines its function, what it will do, and what it can make. Cells live that life, die, are flushed from the body and replaced. But what happens when one group of cells no longer goes along with that plan? This is the case with myeloma, where these plasma cells grow in an abnormal manner and reproduce at a very high rate, thus displacing the healthy cells. So the myeloma patient's bones may be weakened; he loses his normal resistance to disease; he becomes fatigued.

"In Father Greer's case, he told us of what happened in the rectory, and while he didn't really complain, I imagined that he experienced quite severe pain in his back where the myeloma had manifested itself and was still feeling it when he came to us. He lacked that certain vitality that well people have. I tried to be very explicit that he should not take on any more duties at the church and, in fact, try to conserve as much energy as he could so he could best fight this disease. The chemotherapy he would be taking—which attacks the myeloma cells and unfortunately also healthy cells—is strong medication that brings on nausea and alters normal thought patterns. He might tell me on occasion he was a little sick to his stomach, but it was only when I pursued the issue that he would say that he had thrown up. Or thrown up a number of times. He is the kind of patient who, if you forget to ask about a specific side effect, won't bring it up."

Dr. Desforges, during the two years of Father Greer's illness, had seen him many times, for understandably short periods, the average being no more than fifteen or twenty minutes. A lifelong Catholic and a doctor for over forty years, her knowledge of her patient transcended sheer medical expertise, it was soon evident, and it was she, of anyone who knew him, who saw Father Greer most completely. "I think it was especially hard for him because he felt in the prime of his life, a man in charge of his own destiny, and now he wasn't. Father Greer is a gracious man who ministers to others, and suddenly he was the one in need. What worried me about him was that he never called me to unburden himself like most of my patients normally do. In the office he was perfectly logical, answering my questions quietly in a flat voice, signs that he was depressed, and I sensed he was drinking more to compensate. He brought up a priest friend who had died of leukemia and said, 'Look at the two of us.' Father Greer felt the end was in sight, and it took a while for him to realize that he was getting better, that the medicines were working. He was not immediately in danger of dying. I tried to convince him that an illness can have an advantage; patients can cut things out of their lives they don't want to do.

"I tried to impress on him that he should take certain precautions such as wearing a mask on his hospital rounds, and while there was a certain amount of bravado in his refusal, he's not the kind of man who wants to shut himself off from others. I told him repeatedly that he should choose only those things to do that he enjoyed doing. But as I got to know him, it was obvious that being a parish priest is exactly what he wanted to do. He wasn't looking for any excuse to be released from it, even though it was an extremely strenuous job."

I agreed fully with Dr. Desforges, noting my conversation with Father Greer in New Hampshire and his desire to continue indefinitely as a parish priest. I repeated his words: "I see myself functioning as a priest right into my retirement. . . . when I'm retired, I'll want to serve a small parish three or four days a week. With the shortage, I'm sure there'll be a spot for the toddling old Joe Greer."

Dr. Desforges stared at me, her face no longer that of a doctor who obviously cared deeply for a patient, but that of a precise scientist.

"We are making enormous strides in understanding the molecular approaches to cancer treatment," she said. "Over a year ago, here at the medical center, we opened a transplant unit, where formerly fatal diseases of the blood can now be successfully treated by basically killing the bone marrow, replacing it with similar marrow from a donor or the patient's own marrow, which was previously drawn. But myeloma is very, very difficult, seeing that the disease is based in the marrow itself. Someday we hope to use the transplant method on myeloma, but for now . . ."

She took a piece of paper from a desk drawer and, starting at the upper left-hand corner, began to draw a graph. "Thirty to forty percent of myeloma patients don't respond to treatment at all, and they die. These are the rest," she said as the line moved horizontally a third of the way across the page. "In a year, perhaps two or three, it's not unlikely that Father Greer will have a recurrence," she continued as the line dipped, "and he may or may not respond to the second round of treatment. Eventually the body builds up an immunity to the chemotherapy, and the drugs are no longer effective. The myeloma takes over, and there is nothing we can do." Her pencil line moved inexorably downward. "The excess proteins can kill the kidneys and have harmful effects on other organs, or, as is often the case, the patient dies of an infection. The average life span of the myeloma patient, from diagnosis to death, is between two and three years."

Her line had reached the bottom right-hand corner, zero on the chart. "Ten or twelve years would be extraordinary. Quite extraordinary."

I asked if that was the absolute estimate.

"No. There are always exceptions, and with the strides being made, especially in bone marrow transplants, we are always hopeful. Medicine only knows so much and can do so much. Of course, there are other forces that we can never explain. Unexplained—miraculous, if you will—cures occur. But we must also be realistic."

Father Greer had never talked about his illness this way. He had always said it was fatal and incurable, but the way he had said those words had somehow not precisely conveyed their meaning.

I left the New England Medical Center, and instead of driving home as I had planned to do, I was overtaken by a desire to see Father Greer immediately. I didn't know what I wanted to say to him, if anything. As I drove along, I saw before me, as if projected onto the windshield, two graphs: one formed by Father McCarthy's hand as it swooped down over his desk, his dramatic gesture for all the priests who would be lost when the men of Father Greer's era reached their retirement years, the other Dr. Desforges's. And I realized that it was on the physician's diagram that the end of Father Joseph Greer's years as a priest would most likely be recorded.

I arrived at the rectory just as Fathers Greer, Mullaney, and Rossi and Monsignor Mahoney were finishing their supper. I mentioned where I had been, and Father Greer inquired after Dr. Desforges as if I had just visited an old friend or relative of his. Father Greer offered supper: chicken breasts in cream sauce, broccoli, and salad. At a minimum, I had to try a piece of the apple pie Dolly Peters, the evening cook, had made.

Father Greer, sitting at the head of the table, appeared robust and happy. "Those boys are really chipping away at the lower church. What a mess. But they assure me it'll be ready by May. Maybe Mr. Andrew Lane will have his condos up by then and we can get a group rate for blessings when the cardinal comes. Renovated church, house for the homeless, and fancy condos. Same blessing? I'm sure the cardinal can ad-lib one for each. Looks like four hundred thousand smackers for that lower church; let's hope all the good souls of St. Patrick's aren't too put out when all the old statues don't make a resurrection. What do you think?"

The three other priests smiled knowingly.

For once, in the company of Father Greer, which by now was so wonderful and familiar, I found I had nothing to say. I stared dumbly at the pie before me, at the mound of vanilla ice cream melting beside it. I was afraid to raise my head; I was sure my face would tell more than I wanted it to. I finally looked up.

I looked at a man who was, after all, the country priest I had sought.

"By the way," he said, "the hundred-thousand-dollar couple who said they *might* be back?"

I nodded, waiting to hear that they had not and that Father Greer had run into them on the street.

"They're in church every Sunday. And going to Communion. They're even picking out the scripture for their nuptial Mass; they really want to get involved.

"How about that?" he added.

10

*You're not the sort who can talk without saying anything,
and unfortunately that's what's wanted now.*

Father Greer arrives late, as he does for most social events. The hot
and cold hors d'oeuvres are moving nicely, and customers at the
cash bar, set up in the corner of the St. Patrick's school auditorium,
are two deep. The round tables are jammed together, but the crowd
seems not to mind the obstacle course. Others had to be turned
away at the door. Usually Father Greer slips in quietly at such large
gatherings and is gone in less than a half hour, but when he finally
does appear at the side door, he is greeted by applause from a crowd
of some two hundred fifty people.

White doves of peace made of felt, resting on felt olive branches
on pale blue poster board backgrounds, are affixed to the walls and
the stage curtain. CONGRATULATIONS, FATHER GREER reads a huge
banner on one wall, and across the hall two huge blowups of photographs show a handsome twenty-seven-year-old Father Greer in
1958, with a rakish smile, and Father Greer in 1988, at fifty-seven,
standing before a microphone, his posture not as erect, the smile
somewhat faded but still winning. It is a cold winter's night in Natick
and the people of St. Patrick's and other parishes he has served are
here to commemorate that February day thirty years before, when
a young man from Roxbury received, at the hand of Cardinal Cushing, the sacrament of ordination.

Father Greer moves slowly through the crowd, shaking hands,

waving to old friends, allowing the ladies to kiss him on the cheek. He wears a white carnation with a sprig of baby's breath on the lapel of his black jacket.

It is not usual for a priest to be specially honored on the thirtieth anniversary of his ordination, but the Garveys and Barrys and other active St. Patrick's parishioners were not about to let the event pass without doing something. They thought of having a huge private party but were worried that Father Greer might not come. ("Oh, no, you're not," he told Ann Garvey when she mentioned such a party.) They knew if it was a public celebration, he couldn't refuse.

They didn't know that his latest blood counts were good; most of them knew little about the specifics of his illness. They just sensed that they had best do what their hearts told them, regardless of the pastor's recalcitrance. "If something happens soon and we missed this chance to say thank you," said Ann Garvey, "we just wouldn't forgive ourselves."

From a spicy ziti salad to tender sirloin tip steaks, the meal is unusually delicious, given that it is a sit-down affair for so many people. The master of ceremonies, Joseph Keefe, Natick's super-intendent of schools, takes from a book on Thomas Merton a chapter heading, "Among the Shining Vineyards," as the evening's theme and promises to keep on schedule so that Father Greer won't miss his ten o'clock bedtime. Speakers are interspersed between courses of the dinner. Proclamations from the Massachusetts Senate and the Natick selectmen are read, and then the gentle roasting of Father Greer begins. A member of his Boston College class notes that Joe Greer studied business there, with an emphasis in marketing, and that though he could have just as well applied his talents to selling Colgate toothpaste, he chose to work on something more important than people's teeth. Former parishioners puzzle at how he always kept his hair so neat. One reads a poem about Father Greer's jogging days: "He only cried 'Foul' when he heard a growl," an allusion to his well-known dislike for dogs.

Father Greer, who had been seated at a table near the front, does not turn full face to the praise and the benign jibes, preferring to sit facing the wall, offering only a profile to the people on stage. But it is obvious he is enjoying himself; while he looks off to the side much of the time, it is with, if not exactly a smile, a pleased look on his face.

People from the vineyards in which he has labored come and, one after another, tell what he has meant to them. He baptized their children and married many of them. He visited their sick relatives and buried them. He was a man they could always count on. They have had great priests before and since, but there is a special place in their hearts for Father Greer. They miss him. "When my father died, my mother said, 'I've got to get a hold of my friend,' " one former parishioner recalls. "Father Greer was at his next parish, but he came back to say the last rites for the man my mother spent over fifty years of her life with; we'll never forget you for that, Father Joe."

Father Joe. I have never heard him called that, yet tonight there is a depth of intimacy allowed, a gratitude the parishioners want to underscore.

There are so many among them with stories of Father Greer. Scores upon scores are known only to the person affected, and perhaps to their family and close friends. Some are too personal to speak aloud. Like that of the man with the son going bad on drugs whom Father Greer talked to and brought around. Or the family whose teenage daughter he buried with such concern. The woman who attended daily Mass for three decades, unable to receive the Eucharist because of her short, troubled first marriage—it was Father Greer who painstakingly had seen her annulment through the tribunal and wouldn't take no for an answer. The annulment had been granted the week before.

There are nearly a dozen priests there, all except one men of Father Greer's vintage, greying and balding, most with a far more substantial girth than the midsections with which they left St. John's Seminary.

One priest stands out. His long, curling brown hair rests on his shoulders. Although he wears a black suit, his black shirt is open at the neck, where the Roman collar would normally finish off a properly priestly image. His face is innocently young. Yet when he turns a certain way or stands off from the crowd, alone for the moment, the pact is voided and he is Dorian Gray, suddenly old. It is a ravaged face, with soft skin but deep and strangely formed erratic lines on his forehead and chin and cheeks. While he presents a boyish grin throughout his reminiscences of Father Greer, his is a face that has seen and absorbed pain. He is noticeably thin, almost gaunt.

"I was going to get a haircut, but when I knew I was coming tonight, I thought I'd wait a week," Father William Walsh begins. The audience howls and Father Greer rubs his forehead, a broad smile on his face. Father Walsh confesses to being caught in Father Greer's room, a 45 rpm Roy Orbison record blasting out of the stereo, when the pastor returned unexpectedly early one day. He tells about a shaggy dog named Vicar that once sat in Father Greer's favorite lounge chair and left behind so much long hair that Father Greer had to take his suit to the cleaners the next day. "We all know how neat he is," Father Walsh says. "Well, my room was a warehouse. He used to bring people by and say, 'Can you believe there's actually a desk in there somewhere?' He always said if I died in there, he'd never find me and he'd just seal up the room. Well, the day I arrived, hair longer than this, with cowboy boots . . ."

But there is more to Father Walsh's tale—as there probably is to most of the stories told this night.

When Father Walsh called Father Greer in June 1980 to tell him he'd been assigned to St. Joseph's, Hyde Park, he was talking from a residential treatment center for alcoholics. "Joe, look, I'm supposed to come to you, but if you want to get someone else from the diocese, it's okay with me," Father Walsh said. "I'll understand."

Father Greer was not well known to Father Walsh, but the opposite was not true. The personnel office had asked Father Greer to take on the young priest and "straighten him out." While Father Walsh had been a brilliant seminarian, at one time considered for further study in Rome, and a great priest with parish young people, his drinking had gone out of control.

Father Walsh waited for Father Greer's response, ready for a rebuff but hoping it wouldn't come.

Father Greer was not enthusiastic about Walsh being assigned to him, but the clergy personnel director had said he didn't know where to send him or who would accept him. "Try him," the personnel director had pleaded, "and if it gets too bad, call and we'll have him out of there."

"Take your time," Father Greer answered Father Walsh that day. "Get here when you're ready. Don't worry about it."

When Father Walsh arrived, he was given no rules, no preconditions as he expected he might be. Father Greer assigned him duties as he would any other curate. "Billy, here's what you have to do. I'm going to tell you once, and then I'm going to leave you on your own. If you're not doing it, I'll let you know. Otherwise you won't hear from me. And don't expect a lot of pats on the back. I'm not too good at that." What especially struck Father Walsh was that his new pastor never lectured him, never mentioned his drinking problem or told him that what he was doing to or for him was "for your own good." A legion of people had been doing things "for his own good" for years, and now he was an alcoholic. Soon after Father Walsh arrived, he asked to go on vacation, and Father Greer let him go. One Sunday morning during Father Walsh's absence, the pastor was held up at gunpoint. On Father Walsh's return, all Father Greer did was laugh about it.

As Father Walsh would later tell me, talking about his years with Father Greer, "Me, the liberal, and he couldn't have been more a conservative. It didn't look like a good match. But he never said I had to change. He never said I had to cut my hair—and I know it killed him to see me on the altar. He never threatened to kick me out. And he had every reason to do it. In certain ways I was a disgrace. But he could get past the incidentals, as long as I was doing my work. He knew I loved the priesthood; he did, too.

"He's a remarkable man because he's so ordinary. He keeps before him the realization of what we can all be. We get a lot of bad news in our business, but Joe Greer would constantly say we were created to be good. That being your brother's keeper really made sense.

"He realized you can't be all things to all people. But dammit, he tried."

"I was lucky to have some great priests where I grew up in Lowell, men that inspired me, and it's because of them that I became a priest," Father Walsh continues at Father Greer's celebration. "And you, Joe Greer . . ." he says, his voice growing softer.

The St. Patrick's auditorium is still. The other priests are looking down, fiddling with the coffee cups or empty dessert dishes before them. The eyes of the lay audience are fixed on the stage and the thin man in black, his face, while serious, now young and guileless.

". . . you. We all have things to thank Father Greer for tonight. I do too. Joe Greer," he says, looking at the priest, "you're the reason I'm still a priest today. Thanks for believing in me."

Father Walsh comes down from the stage and toward Father Greer and reaches down to give him a hug, which Father Greer accepts uncomfortably.

"Now would you get a haircut?" Father Greer says.

"Joe, for you I will," he says. Tears are streaming down his face.

II

We preserve. No doubt. But we only preserve in order to save, and the world can never realize that, for the world asks only to survive.

The big man with a full head of white hair, dressed in scarlet from his stiff collar to the hem of his garment, which touches the top of his soft black loafers, startles Dolly Peters when he appears at the kitchen door of St. Patrick's rectory on a sunny April afternoon.

"Your—your—"

"Well, hello, and what's your name?" he asks.

"Dolly—Dolly Peters, your—your—"

"Is Father Greer about? I hear we have a beautiful church to dedicate and a house for the homeless. He was kind enough to ask me to come out and give him a hand on this wonderful day. I hear you'll have a bite for us after. What will it be? Something smells very good already."

Bernard Cardinal Law stands in the middle of the kitchen, an imposing, stately man, broad-shouldered and over six feet tall. He seems to be at home immediately, although it is his first visit to St. Patrick's since Father Greer was appointed pastor. It is as if he has just happened by and not that he is here for an afternoon Father Greer has been working toward for years and planning for months. An afternoon that has caused him, normally unflappable pastor that he is, to be at wit's end all week with details from the terrazzo floor in the sacristy (the sealant had dried with a spotty, glutinous sheen and had to be redone) to the rubber mats (they had not arrived) to the light above the statue of Mary (it was hitting her squarely in the back of the neck).

The "bite" the cardinal is referring to is a dinner for the twelve attending priests that Dolly and two other cooks have been working on since early this morning. A long table has been moved into the parlor, the best linens and china employed; a full bar has been set up.

Cardinal Law has been criticized by a good number of his priests for his uncollegial administrative decisions and policy and his unblinking fealty to Rome (among certain priests of the archdiocese he is commonly referred to as "the pope's clone"), but in person he is a consummate and quite accessible statesman. At the dedication of the house for the homeless, he sits in the large common room with some of the residents, commenting appreciatively on the comfortable chairs and sofa and the large television set. He asks where they come from and what they had for breakfast.

With none of them is he overly specific or prying or in any way condescending regarding their current state of affairs. He saves his reflections on their circumstances for his short talk after liberally sprinkling the house with holy water and pronouncing an extemporaneous blessing. (Such places are outside the purview of prayer books, which deal with more ordinary sites.) "What do we do when life deals us a situation we're not happy with? Something we don't think we can take? It's so hard. It seems so hopeless. Yet isn't there always someone, or someplace, that seems to come along that just seems to give us the boost we need so we can get through another day, or make that change that starts to turn things around? This is such a place. I know these walls are clean, but they have love and hope written all over them."

He ends, a bit incongruously, chanting several rounds of the rousing civil rights standard "A-a-men, a-men, amen."

In the sacristy, before the blessing of the lower church, he talks to the altar boys, placing his red skullcap in turn on each head, telling them of his need for priests, and promising, "Now if you come up for pope, remember I get a vote. You'll get mine; you can count on that."

As he did in the house for the homeless, Father Greer stands off to the side, allowing the cardinal center stage. Father Greer, the advance man, does his work so well he is hardly noticed. His interactions with his superior are mostly through whispers and subtle hand gestures, informing him who he should greet, then moving him toward the appropriate door or alb or staircase.

Cardinal Law celebrates the regularly scheduled 5:30 P.M. Mass in the upper church, which is filled almost to capacity. His sermon, delivered without notes, is a potpourri of his travels (he had just returned from Atlanta and the consecration of America's first black archbishop), his congratulations to the parishioners for making possible both a home for the less fortunate and a new place of worship, and finally his praise of Father Greer.

"When I was talking over at the residence about life dealing you something you didn't think you could bear, my mind was on you, Father Greer. What a precious gift life is. And oh, so fragile. A friend of mine died of multiple sclerosis, and near the end he had no speech. He could only hope in silence in the Lord, and I know that's what he did. So death, where is your sting? Whether we live or die, we are the Lord's. It is our hope that transforms us, our hope not in our own abilities or that the situation will change, but hope in the Lord, who will never abandon us.

"And here we are today, people of hope, people of St. Patrick's, people who have in Father Greer a great pastor and a great priest. He faces a terrible disease, and we see the magnificent grace that he faces it with while—"

The applause starts as a gentle ripple near the back of the church and sweeps forward. People rise from the pews. Cardinal Law stops in midsentence and joins in their applause. Father Greer looks out to his people. His hand moves in a slight waving motion for them to stop, but they will not. He shifts uneasily in his chair. He raises both hands in the air, accepting their acclaim.

"—a terrible disease. But," the cardinal continues once the applause is quieted, "here is a man with faith in God, faith in . . ."

On his most recent monthly visits to the New England Medical Center, Father Greer had been noting to Drs. Desforges and Erban that the back pain—the precursor of his disease some two years before—had been recurring. He said it was worse than ever. And that his fatigue was becoming so pronounced he had trouble getting out of bed in the morning and often had to take a nap after lunch. Their physical examinations of Father Greer as well as blood tests indicated the myeloma was still quiescent, and they continued to attribute the pain to a mild arthritis in the area. They told him his fatigue was not directly related to his disease and, as he was not anemic and his blood counts were within a normal range, it was the burden of his job that was wearing him down. Nonetheless, while their examinations and tests showed Father Greer to be in remission, they began to anticipate the next step in his treatment.

As the cardinal's firm voice continues to echo in St. Patrick's upper church, I recall the question Dr. Erban had raised when I visited the medical center alone one day recently: "Are these subjective feelings of fatigue in a man who knows he has an incurable disease? It's very hard to say. Anxiety can cause many symptoms. And while we are making tremendous strides in understanding the biology of blood diseases and the technology for treatment is advancing very quickly, it isn't enough to tell a patient like Father Greer that we are going to know so much more in a year. He knows he might not have that year. Emotionally, we have to offer a plan. When you see—as we have seen recently—Father Greer's increasing lethargy, some evidence of a building depression, and then hear him say that his parish work is 'becoming a chore,' you must offer him something. Not a pipe dream, of course, but the best possible course of treatment. He is not a man comfortable with watching and waiting. Honestly, I can't blame him. It's easy for us to say 'Let's see how this goes and we'll evaluate it next month.' That month is an eternity for the patient."

Father Greer's chemotherapy had been stopped in December. While his doctors had no way of knowing how long the myeloma would stay in remission, they knew they had to be ready once it reappeared—as it almost certainly would. The normal second course of treatment for a multiple myeloma patient such as Father Greer is essentially a repeat of the first: large doses of the drugs prednisone and Alkeran or melphalan. The treatment has remained virtually unchanged since it was perfected some fifteen years ago. Sometimes the second treatment with the powerful drugs succeeds in bringing about another remission; eventually, however, a point is reached when the drugs cannot contain the disease or their toxicity is more than the patient can endure.

Dr. Desforges had informed Father Greer a month before that she was willing—if he was—to try another approach. A bone marrow transplant.

She and Dr. Erban had explained the procedure, underscoring the possibility that the treatment itself could kill him but also holding out the hope—slim as it was—that a transplant might rid him of myeloma. Normally, a transplant for multiple myeloma would not be attempted on a patient over fifty years of age, but because Father Greer's physical condition was that of a thirty-five-year-old, they felt he could withstand the treatment. They were also impressed with his mental stability and the apparently deep reservoir of his spiritual life. "The mind must be able to withstand this as well as the body," Dr. Desforges had told him.

Father Greer was scheduled for the battery of psychological tests that are given to prospective transplant patients to ascertain their personality traits and the likelihood of their sustaining the post-transplant isolation as well as the pain and trauma of the long recovery period. He would also be subjected to a detailed screening to assess every possible medical particular, from the state of his teeth to his propensity to contract herpes. Bleeding gums or a herpes infection, for the normally healthy person annoyances that are easily treated, can be fatal to the posttransplant patient.

"We want the lowest possible risk with the greatest possibility of return," Dr. Desforges said on one visit, and Father Greer chided her for sounding like an investment banker. "It's hard to know exactly when the best time is, so the best we can do now is wait," she told him. "And I know that is hard, but we don't want to move until it is prudent to do so. For now, the disease is behaving itself. After all, perhaps no more than twenty-five people have been transplanted for myeloma; the follow-up time is short, no more than a year or two; we don't know exactly why it works better in some cases and less well in others. We have so little information. And so we are planning for the future. You are listed as a transplant candidate, and while you will be making all the preparations, for now you are on hold."

Because of those preparations, Father Greer began to make more frequent trips into Boston—now driving a new Mercury Cougar with a plush maroon interior that he had impulsively bought off the showroom floor one afternoon. "The most luxurious car I ever owned," he noted. He saw no special significance in the fact that he had bought that type of car at the time he did.

The back pain persisted, and Father Greer continued to complain to his doctors of increasing fatigue and sleeplessness. His doctors told him to take painkillers or sleeping pills as needed and to please try to work less, "to save a few less souls," as Dr. Desforges put it. Father Greer shrugged off both suggestions. He did not want "to become addicted to pills," and as for church work, "I don't have any choice. One of my priests is looking for a new assignment; I've been through three custodians this year; marriages are pouring in, and each one requires five appointments. Save souls? That's a joke. I went over for a visit to our CCD classes and talked to the kids. 'You go to church, honey?' I asked this little third-grade girl. 'No, Mommy has to go to aerobics.' I asked another one. 'No, Mommy works and she has to sleep on weekends.' That's the level I'm on. My spiritual director tells me I should make up a calendar of what I do each day, so I can get a better idea of how I spend my time. I don't have time to do that either."

"It's very important to take time for yourself," Dr. Erban told him. "Physically, you are fit. Mentally, you have to be prepared if we are to do the transplant."

"Let me put that on my list," Father Greer responded with a small smile as he sat on the examining table, slumped over more wearily than usual. " 'Get mentally prepared.' "

"We are grateful for Father Greer," the cardinal goes on, making good on his promise to Father Greer to deliver a sermon so long he may never be asked back to St. Patrick's. "We sense the presence of the risen Christ in him, and he knows he is in our thoughts and in our prayers. Father Greer, our hats are off to you for what you have done here at St. Patrick's."

After Mass, the two men walk from the church through the covered passageway leading to the rectory, the cardinal with his arm over the priest's shoulder. The general and the field lieutenant, an officer who had been sent to a difficult post and delivered in the finest tradition of the corps. The cardinal goes on about the enthusiasm of the people, the beauty of the lower church, the outreach provided by the house for the homeless.

Father Greer nods but demurs. He hasn't done that much, he says. It was the generosity of the people who provided the funds and good craftsmen who completed the work. They go into the rectory for dinner.

There is something else on Father Greer's mind, something he was informed of earlier this week. Being a master of timing, he knows this, the end of a happy day, is not the right moment to tell the cardinal. It can be done later, in a letter or a call to the cardinal's secretary.

His myeloma has returned. The chemotherapy has kept it at bay for less than five months.

I had spent the better part of a year with Father Greer, watching him at work and eventually hearing him talk about himself and the life of a parish priest. His illness had been relegated to the background.

Now, with the return of the multiple myeloma and the decision of the doctors at New England Medical Center to proceed with a radical treatment—a bone marrow transplant—it was at the forefront.

Father Greer was in as good a physical condition as he might ever hope to be, given that he had a fatal disease. If the second round of chemotherapy worked as the doctors hoped it would, the myeloma could be kept at a low level for some months. Dr. Desforges asked Father Greer for the best time for the transplant to take place, given the long recuperative period it would demand, and he said the early fall. He wanted it no earlier as, in addition to his parish work, he was planning a full summer of golf and a trip—his ninth—to visit his cousins in Ireland. He also wanted to play golf in Scotland on the way back.

Backdating from the middle of September, Dr. Desforges began scheduling more frequent visits to the New England Medical Center clinics and hospital. As Father Greer was to receive not an allogeneic transplant, where a genetically alike donor contributes marrow, but an autologous transplant in which his own blood cells would be extracted, frozen, and later returned to him, the preparation would require a minimum of three months.

Father Greer notified the Boston Archdiocese of the transplant date and the fact that he would be convalescing for at least six months afterward. He offered to resign his pastorate or to be transferred.

A year before I had gone looking for a "country priest," a man facing death. I had found Father Greer and had gladly abandoned my search.

Now, after all, I had my country priest.

Sadly, it was Father Greer.

Part 2

I

What lay behind me was no longer any normal, familiar life, that everyday life out of which the impulse to pray raises us, with still at the back of our minds the certainty that whatsoever we wish we can return. A void was behind me. And in front a wall, a wall of darkness.

On the right or north side of Kneeland Street, as it travels west from the harbor toward Boston Common, is a decaying yet vibrant neighborhood made up of squat, undistinguished old buildings. This is Boston's Chinatown—with its gaudy restaurants and shops and crowded apartments—and also Boston's Combat Zone, where shabby signs promise sensual delights.

On the left side of Kneeland are a group of taller, more subdued buildings of varying heights and ages, vaguely uniform in their shades of chalky beige: the New England Medical Center. Urban redevelopment, which in the last two decades has placed a premium on this property so close to downtown, promises gradually to swallow up the porn shows and shops and the bars, as well as the small but affordable apartments and less successful Chinese merchants on the north side of Kneeland. Across the street medical science and human need have prevailed, even as real estate prices soared. The New England Medical Center, and the Tufts Medical and Dental schools within it, has grown both through new construction and by leap-frogging into nearby existing buildings, creating a labyrinth of hallways, stairwells, and ramps that has necessitated the building of covered passageways to span streets and connect structures converted to hospital use. Amid this array of buildings there is one especially startling flying passageway that bridges Washington Street. Painted a brilliant red, it gives the appearance of a huge artery connecting two organs that require its size and robustness.

New England Medical Center is called a "primary referral center," which means that it accepts many patients who require the specialized attention or treatment unavailable in local hospitals. Currently, it has 480 beds, 364 for adults and 116 for children. Founded in 1796, it is the oldest hospital in New England, third oldest in the nation, and one that long has had a reputation for both excellent patient care and medical research. It was at the center that the link between obesity and heart disease was proved and where the fundamental research was done that led to the discovery of a drug that suppresses the immune reaction and thus allows organs to be transplanted into a recipient body, which normally would reject them. The first laser heart surgery was performed here, and recently interleukin-2 was used as an innovative treatment for cancer. Hematology—the specialty dealing with blood disorders and the medical discipline under which Father Greer is being treated— was virtually born at the center with the pioneering work of Dr. William Damashek in the 1930s. New England Medical Center ranks sixth in the nation in National Institutes of Health grants and is the first choice of many medical students who apply for residencies and fellowships in such fields as cardiology, neurology, newborn medicine, and hematology and oncology, which is considered to be a dual specialty including both blood diseases and cancers.

Back in the late 1960s, when Father Greer was assigned to St. James the Greater parish, only a block from Kneeland, Chinatown and the Combat Zone were by far the dominant presences on Kneeland Street, the medical center a respected but small institution housed in only three buildings. His assignment as the chaplain of the center's pediatric ward—called "The Floating" after a hospital ship for children that had once been moored in Boston Harbor— led him to sound one of the few retreats in his priesthood. "I'd go in and see those kids, so many of them dying, try to say something to their parents," he said as we walked through the third-floor waiting area in The Floating one morning, "and it was just wiping me out. Every once in a while, I'd find myself sitting in a bar across Kneeland in the middle of the afternoon, drinking beer, eating peanuts, and throwing the shells on the floor. I don't even like beer. I asked for a reassignment."

He looked neither to the right nor to the left as we passed through the third floor of The Floating on his way to Biewend 3. Later he claimed he could not hear the cries issuing from the young patients there.

Since the time he had been brought to the center by ambulance two years before, its clinics, labs, and hallways had become all too familiar to him. Proger, Tupper, Biewend, Ziskind, Pratt, Farnsworth are all buildings he can easily navigate. But by far it is the room with rose-colored walls in Biewend 3, the hematology/oncology clinic, that he knows best.

While the New England Medical Center is considered to be at the forefront of medical knowledge and treatment, an institution anyone afflicted with serious disease would be fortunate to be treated at, it does not give off (like a general hospital, with its maternity floors and dozens of routine operations for inflamed tonsils and ruptured appendices and disks) that unquantifiable feeling of a facility where patients enter in pain or need and leave repaired or cured, generally on their way to good health. It is not that the medical center is grim, for it is not; the receptionists are for the most part polite and patient, the nurses and doctors are hardly glum, the surroundings are airy, brightly painted, and well maintained.

Yet in the waiting rooms and hallways, in the cafeteria, even in the parking garage, there are so many faces—stricken, numb faces—conveying unfathomable grief.

While Father Greer's usual visits to the medical center take no more than an hour and a half, he was aware that that day he would spend all morning. The date for his transplant was less than a month away. He had passed the psychological screening and had gone through a series of complex preparations over the past two months. During this last month, the procedures would be even more involved. A number of the items on the check-off sheet he had been given early in the summer had to be addressed that day, before he would be able to phone his friend, Father James Canniff, to pick him up and take him back to St. Mary's rectory in Charlestown, where his car was parked.

The new hematology fellow assigned to his case, Dr. Rebecca Shulman,* did the initial physical examination on Father Greer and checked the results of his blood counts. Dr. Shulman, a small, intense woman with short-cropped hair, was quite unlike Dr. John Erban, whom she replaced. Dr. Shulman was not given to small talk or personal conversation, as was Dr. Erban, and Father Greer sat quietly while she slowly passed the stethoscope back and forth over his chest and rib cage and along his back.

Father Greer had grown to like the easy familiarity of Dr. Erban, and Dr. Erban had grown to understand him. "So many patients rely on you, and it's very flattering as a young doctor—until they begin to die on you and you feel your guts torn out," Dr. Erban said, recalling his relationship with the priest. "But with Father Greer, while I knew he appreciated what I did and he wanted to be cured, I never felt he depended on me. Doctors were not his only chance. He was always a pleasure to see. He didn't bring in a burden and lay it on my shoulders." In July, when the medical fellows were rotated, Dr. Erban had left to do research within the medical center. Father Greer found Dr. Shulman to be Dr. Erban's opposite, and personally less compatible. He answered all the questions she asked of him but did not offer much of his usual banter, which he sensed was now unwelcome.

For Dr. Shulman, it was an equally uncomfortable association. Father Greer was the first patient she had seen on her first day in clinic. He was a priest, already somewhat a mystery to her, a religious Jew, and she sensed that being treated by a young woman might make him feel ill at ease. As a result she displayed even more reserve with him than she ordinarily did.

And there was something else. Her own father had been diagnosed with multiple myeloma shortly before she had arrived for her fellowship. Thoughts of him would flood into her mind as she examined Father Greer or asked him the series of routine questions on each visit—questions she was now asking her own father—but she quickly drove them away. Her own mental exertion undoubtedly made her seem more abrupt and clinical.

While Dr. Shulman was noting her findings, Dr. Desforges entered the room. As usual, she had a ready smile and a warm "Good morning, Father Greer." She continued, "I hear you took a trip up to your place in New Hampshire. That's wonderful. Just the thing to do. Get away when you can. You're looking pretty fit for a man we've been sticking with needles and extracting all sorts of things from. Your white count is up, so the mild doses of chemotherapy you're taking are doing their job. I'm glad to hear that you're tolerating the medicine better; the stomach has settled down, hasn't it? Everything is looking just fine for the transplant. There's a bit of a backup with the isolation rooms, so I'm sorry to say that we have to delay your transplant a few weeks, until later in September, but that shouldn't bother anything. How are you feeling?"

"Pretty good, pretty good. The ribs are still a little sore over here," he said flatly as he touched a point low on the right side, "where the pneumonia dropped in to pay a visit. I get tired quicker than I should. Not sleeping the best. The pneumonia?" He appeared to slouch at the sound of the word as if he were trapped in an elevator shaft and the elevator was being let down a few inches at a time. "Is that . . . well . . . going to stand in the way?"

Dr. Shulman reported there was just the slightest indication of fluid in his lungs, and Dr. Desforges reexamined his chest and back before repeating what she had told Father Greer on the two previous visits: that his resistance was lower and pneumonia was almost predictable because myeloma cells crowd out the normal, healthy white blood cells that fight infection. But in answer to his question, no: the transplant was still on. Dr. Desforges stood back, looking at Father Greer's form, slumped over as he balanced on the edge of the examining table.

"Anything going on that I should know?"

Father Greer paused. The doctors waited. "This old thing up here," he said, pointing to his head, "keeps buzzing around. Can't get through a night. Wondering. It's hard to believe I'm as sick as I am, feeling as good as I do. Say, what kind of shape am I going to be in when I get out of here, anyhow?"

"When you get *out*," Dr. Desforges said brightly, emphasizing the word, "you'll feel crummy, out of shape, but soon after, you should begin to feel reasonably okay. The body takes a while to recoup. We think of a year as the normal time it takes a person to really recover. Here in the hospital, we'll be very careful of your diet until your immune system kicks in—a little bug on a leaf of lettuce could cause you distress, so we'll be cooking and serving your food very carefully—and for a while after you're released you must watch out, but soon your diet will pretty much be back to normal. Usually within a hundred days your marrow should be producing all the blood cells you need. The big difference in your kind of transplant is that your own marrow doesn't fight you when we give it back."

"We're on speaking terms. I hope," Father Greer added with a small smile.

"Far more important than the pneumonia or your diet is your mental state. It's very important for you to understand everything that's going to happen and not to hesitate to ask questions or to call any of us at any time with whatever is on your mind. You know you can do that, don't you?"

He nodded and said nothing. Dr. Desforges hesitated, once again leaving a conversational vacuum, something most patients would fill. But Father Greer did not. As the transplant date neared, she was growing concerned that none of Father Greer's friends or family members had contacted her about the procedure, its side effects, and his chances and that the priest himself had rarely contacted her outside of normal visits.

"We feel very positive about this, Father; we're using the very latest technique, the one that really holds out great promise. Two years ago it wouldn't have been possible. We're learning so quickly about your disease and transplants. But you also understand what we will put you through. I don't want to gloss that over."

He had been told many times. The massive doses of chemotherapy and X rays would, in effect, kill him. His bone marrow would be wiped out and with it the body's capacity to produce blood cells. He would experience constant nausea and severe diarrhea. Open sores would erupt in his mouth and throughout his gastrointestinal system. He would lose his hair, have painfully swollen glands, and perhaps suffer from hallucinations. The procedure would sterilize him, and in all probability he would eventually develop cataracts. He would experience high fevers. A bone marrow transplant is considered the "rescue" from this medically inflicted death, but if the transplant failed to engraft and his marrow did not produce healthy cells, he could die of an infection or internal bleeding. He could go into cardiac arrest or kidney failure because of the drugs.

"I understand." He buttoned up his shirt.

Drs. Desforges and Shulman turned to leave.

"By the way . . . I heard about John Andrews," said Father Greer.

"Let's hope for the best out in Seattle," said Dr. Desforges.

When Father Greer returned to the waiting area, Terry Fogaran was there waiting for him, a clipboard under her arm. An ebullient, noticeably pregnant woman in her mid-twenties, she was the transplant unit's coordinator. It was her responsibility to ensure that the patient knew everything about the procedure, met all the people who would be involved, and saw each of the places where treatment would be performed.

After going over a small list of routine items Father Greer was to bring into the hospital, such as robes, comfortable pajamas, and slippers, she said, "Also pictures, photographs of nice scenes, loved ones, books you like, anything pleasant to connect you to the outside world. You'll be in isolation, and you want the room to be as cheery as possible. Maybe a calendar?"

"Like I'm doing time?" Father Greer said as we wound our way through The Floating and into Proger.

"I understand. Whatever is good for you. I'd bring anything I'd want if I knew I would be stuck in a room for six weeks."

"I've got the archdiocesan CCD people sending me a bunch of videotapes on social justice and prayer," he said. "Might as well do a miniretreat while I'm in; we're supposed to do one every year, and I'm due. I'll bring my Mass kit. Is that all right?"

"You might find the wine a bit irritating to the stomach in the early days, but sure, bring it along. There'll be a refrigerator in the room, so you can have food anytime you can eat it."

"I won't be much for that, will I?"

"No, the appetite is pretty suppressed, at least in the early stages. Most of your nutrition will be given intravenously until you can drink and eat. Here we are; have you been on Six North before?"

Proger 6 North looks little different from many hospital wards. It has a main nurses' station, open on all sides, and narrow hallways filled with the necessities of hospital life: wheelchairs, mobile linen racks, portable blood pressure gauges, warming bins from the last meal. The difference would be apparent only to the practiced medical eye. The rooms have double metal cabinets, one over the other, next to the door, which has a large glass window. And there is a twenty-four-hour pharmacy located on the floor.

Both hematology and oncology patients are treated here: people suffering from various cancers of the marrow and blood—leukemias, lymphomas, and multiple myeloma—as well as those with solid-tumor cancers of the breast, lung, brain, and internal organs and those with aplastic anemia. On a status board behind the desk area the names of the hematology patients are written on blue tape, those of the oncology patients on yellow.

Terry stopped at room 664.

"Everything coming into the room will be passed through these," she said, touching the cabinet doors, "which will reduce the chance of infection. Your nurse and those three or four people who will be allowed to visit you will scrub and wear masks, gowns, and rubber gloves. You'll have your own TV, VCR, and an intercom so we can eliminate as much traffic in and out as possible. The room is designed so that there is a pressure built up inside; air is constantly being pushed out. It's being prepared for the next patient, so we can visit."

Room 664 was twelve by sixteen feet with a partial divider, waist high, a third of the way in. There was a small private bathroom. On the ceiling over the bed was a huge NuAire air filter. The view out the window was to the back of some brick buildings a bit to the east. The walls were a restful green and the metal of the bed railings and the IV poles that stood at the head of the bed looked new.

"There are two rooms which we use for transplant patients," Terry said as we left. "The patient next door in six sixty-five is about five days posttransplant." The door to 665 was closed, the shade drawn.

"The worst time," Father Greer said.

"Yes, it is," she replied.

After a visit to the dietitian, who outlined the foods he should avoid once he was released (such as raw vegetables, home-baked goods, and anything which has not been either thoroughly cooked or commercially packaged), Father Greer thanked Terry for her help and walked up the stairs to the blood bank on the eighth floor. The nurses and technicians looked pleased to see him, and he them.

"How about the middle of September for our cruise?" Father Greer said. "My buddy Bobby Devereaux has this forty-six-footer; we'll sail over to Plymouth for lunch. How does that sound to you folks?"

"Great," said Lisa Jueppner. "And I got that videotape on hold for you as soon as you come in."

"And which is that, my dear?"

"*Dirty Dancing*, Father, how could you forget?"

"*Dirty Dancing?*"

"I was doing anything I could to keep you awake while we had you in captivity. If you liked the music—as they say—you'll *love* the movie."

Father Greer's eyes scanned the cluster of three orange lounge chairs, each with an IV pole attached, passed over the emaciated figure of a young man receiving a transfusion in one of the chairs, and then took in the two rooms at the rear, each outfitted with chair, bed, and a console that sat on top of what looked like a small washing machine.

"I can hardly wait."

Father Greer had spent five to six hours in one of these rooms during each of the eight visits he had made here over the past two months. An intravenous needle had extracted blood from a vein in one arm and another needle had returned it to the opposite arm after the blood had passed through the newest of the blood bank's pheresis machines, a Fenwal CS-3000. Through the simple working of centrifugal force, his B-positive blood was separated in a bell-shaped glass receptacle called a Latham bowl. The heavier red blood cells were thrust to the outside, while the white blood cells formed a thin band of a viscous liquid, which was continually siphoned off into a four-by-eight-inch rectangular plastic bag strung above him on an IV pole. Within this pink, cloudy liquid were a group of peripheral stem cells, cells medical science has long known about yet has never seen, cells that were Father Greer's hope for a cure from his otherwise fatal disease.

Peripheral stem cells, immature cells that occur predominantly in the marrow, are the building blocks of the blood from which red and white cells as well as platelets are derived. While most stem cells circulate and eventually incubate in the marrow, some remain in the body's bloodstream—the periphery—and travel with the mature white blood cells until they are needed back in the marrow to produce a new generation of cells. For every one thousand to ten thousand white cells, there is a single peripheral stem cell, or so researchers believe. As stem cells have never been isolated and therefore cannot be tracked, their presence can only be assumed until they have begun to mature.

All of the body's blood—some five thousand cubic centimeters, more than five quarts—is circulated through the leukopheresis machine every hour, and to prevent the veins from collapsing from the slight suction the process involves, the patient is instructed to keep kneading a small foam rubber rectangle. Blood bank personnel like Lisa and Carole Gross and Allen Smith are responsible for keeping the patient awake and flexing, whatever prodding, impetus, or provocation is required.

During one of his leukopheresis appointments, Father Greer had finally met John Andrews, to whom he was intimately linked though who up to now had been only a name.

Andrews was the other multiple myeloma patient undergoing leukopheresis in preparation for a transplant. Father Greer was amazed by Andrews's healthy appearance and effervescent manner. "He looked like a well-tanned golf pro," Father Greer said. "He said he had some pain, but never got tired. I was tired all the time. He was thirty-seven; I had twenty years on him. I couldn't figure it out: he had a count in the high teens on his blood protein, mine was only seven. That meant he was a lot sicker than I was, but he looked great. We both knew that if his protein got too high, they would scratch him for a transplant. But he said, 'I'm going to beat it.' "

"We're both going to beat it," Father Greer had replied.

By the middle of July—just before Father Greer's intended trip to Ireland—eight sacks containing the peripheral stem cells had been diluted with a preservative called dimethylsulfoxide, or DMSO, frozen, and placed in a waist-high tank of liquid nitrogen that would keep them at minus 400 degrees Fahrenheit. After Father Greer's last visit to the blood bank, Dr. Kenneth Miller, the head of the New England Medical Center bone marrow transplant unit and a man who had been trained as a resident fellow by Dr. Desforges, had had the priest admitted and brought to the operating room. There, with Father Greer under general anesthetic and with the sound track from *The Big Chill* playing—most doctors in the OR work to music—he had made some hundred insertions with a four-inch-long hypodermic needle high on Father Greer's hips and removed about a thousand cubic centimeters of marrow from his pelvis. This, too, had been frozen.

Within a week Father Greer was free to travel to Ireland.

While Father Greer had never been to continental Europe or felt the desire to travel to Rome, the seat of Catholicism, this was his ninth trip to Ireland. He wanted to visit once again the tiny village of Castlebar, County Mayo, this time to allay the fears of the McDonalds and the Larkins, his relatives on his mother's side, who had heard of his illness through family in the States. "I wanted them to see me, who, for reasons beyond my understanding, they regard as their favorite nephew," he explained to me upon his return. "I guess it's because of the priesthood. When I pulled up in the car, they came out and gave me that warm Irish greeting: 'You're welcome; you're very welcome; you're most welcome.' These wonderful people who have such a hard life. They still burn peat, and my Aunt Kate, who is seventy-eight, still milks ten cows by hand every day. But the spirit they have! They said they'd been praying for me. But they're practical. 'What be the odds, Father?' they asked.

"So I explained the bone marrow transplant to them—of course, they had never heard of such a thing—and told them the odds must be pretty good or else I wouldn't have been selected for a transplant in the first place. I said a private Mass for them at the local church, got a couple of quarts of Johnny Powers whiskey—coarse as sandpaper, but they love it—spent a hundred bucks or so on a nice spread of food, and we all had a wonderful evening together. I told them to keep on praying for me, but not to worry, I'd be back next June for aunt's fiftieth wedding anniversary.

" 'We'll be waiting,' they said.

"That anything should happen, God forbid, I wanted that visit. And then there was the other reason for the trip: a few rounds of golf on one of the world's most beautiful courses, Gleneagles in Perth.

"By the time we [he was traveling with three priest friends, James

Canniff, Edward Sviokla, and Paul White] got to Scotland, I was feeling pretty bum. I had tremendous headaches, and headaches are something I never get. I was aching all over, and there was a pain in my chest that wouldn't go away. I couldn't swing a golf club without it just about killing me, so I checked into a hospital in Perth. The doctors were shocked to find out I was a transplant candidate. My white blood count was way down. I had pneumonia.

"Something happened at the hospital. When I went in for my X rays, I took off my shirt and a nice gold cross and chain the Hajjars had given me. When I came out, the shirt was there, but the cross was stolen. A teachable moment, as we say in moral philosophy, but what was I being taught?

"The doctors in Perth wanted me to get on a plane and get back to the States right away. But I didn't want to ruin the vacation for the other guys."

Father Greer spent over a week in his hotel room at Gleneagles. It embarrassed him how his friends looked after him. They brought him meals; they didn't seem that interested in going out to play golf, for which they had traveled almost three thousand miles. It was still another testament of the fellowship between priests, especially on the part of Father Canniff. A burly, barrel-chested man, a rapid-fire talker who whizzes through his Masses in two thirds the time it takes a meticulous man like Father Greer, Father Canniff was in many ways his opposite. Yet in other ways they were very much alike: neither would describe himself as an especially empathetic or patient type, espousing instead the priestly style of their era—rough-and-ready generalists, able to handle with equanimity and dispatch leaking pipes, a funeral, the late arrival of Easter flowers, or the reluctance of parishioners to shoulder their fiscal responsibilities. Neither would—or did—talk about their innermost feelings or spiritual life to each other. And yet there was a bond. Whenever Father Canniff would pick up his friend after a grueling chemotherapy session at the New England Medical Center, glance across the front seat, and say, "Rough one, huh, Joe?" Father Greer felt the kind of uninvasive compassion he could easily accept.

"I had a lot of time to think in Perth," Father Greer said as we talked in his room at St. Patrick's. "And I'm afraid to admit I lapsed. I went into a mental nosedive. The myeloma cells were growing rapidly, pushing out the white cells; I knew it for sure. My body was filling up with cancer.

"I had gone through all the tedious preparation for the transplant only to get pneumonia and wash out. I knew the transplant was my only chance, and a long shot at that, for any kind of long-term remission, and now it looked like I'd be too sick to withstand it. I knew what it involved. I knew that a percentage die just from the procedure or from an infection when their blood didn't regenerate. But when you face a slow death or the slimmest possibility of a cure, what would anybody do? Now even that hope was being taken away.

"I knew the physical danger, the psychological danger, and in Scotland I came face to face, once again and this time stronger than ever, with the spiritual danger. I was abandoning hope. Faith? Very far away, faith.

"I had these tortured monologues:

" 'I'm a good guy, God; why are You doing this to me?'

" 'Why are You punishing me like this?'

" 'I've tried, You know I've tried, to do my job; is this my reward? More of a cross than I can bear.'

"As with any one-way conversation, I wasn't giving the other party a chance to reply. I wasn't open for a reply, anyhow. I was sullen, depressed; I couldn't figure out why God was picking on me. At times like that a man can get angry at God, and I guess I was angry. I was feeling very sorry for myself."

2

How little we know what a human life really is—even our own. To judge us by what we call our actions is probably as futile as to judge us by our dreams. God's justice chooses from this dark conglomeration of thought and act, and that which is raised toward the Father shines with a sudden burst of light, displayed in glory like the sun.

Pneumonia struck once more, and the Archdiocese of Boston finally spoke. The invasion of Father Greer's lungs and his release from the pastorate of St. Patrick's occurred within days of each other in late August.

As the summer progressed, Father Greer did not exactly welcome a first and then a second postponement of his transplant date. But he was not unduly dismayed. After all, the archdiocese had still not appointed the interim administrator, something the personnel office had promised to do even before Father Greer left for Ireland in July. And while he was a transplant candidate who had to be in Boston one, two, or even three days a week, he was still a full-time pastor of an enormous church with an understaffed rectory. Also, the delays allowed him to rationalize that there were those more needy of a transplant than he. In a strange way, the delays he read as good signs.

By the time the chancery finally decided on his replacement and the new man was due to arrive, that had all changed. Father Greer had become consumed with the desire to get on with the transplant.

Procedurally, he wanted to observe priestly etiquette—not to be in residence as the lame-duck pastor—but personally, he was frightened. The illness in Scotland had alarmed him; a further bout of pneumonia in August that had necessitated an emergency three-day stay at Leonard Morse Hospital in Natick (it was a weekend, and there were no beds available at New England Medical Center) filled him with morbid foreboding. His myeloma was active, that he knew, and as he spent one restless night after another, he convinced himself that the disease was rampaging through his body. His time was running out.

During the week in September when the last of the check-off items was addressed and he was "fitted" for radiation—contorted into a fetal position with his arms taped to his sides and his knees thrust up to his face, then unceremoniously stuffed into the diamond-shaped box that would contain him while his entire body was blasted with lethal amounts of radiation—Father Greer heard that John Andrews had "washed out" of the transplant program. The New England Medical Center transplant team of doctors had determined that because of Andrews's continually rising protein count, his myeloma was too advanced for their procedure to work. The Fred Hutchinson Center in Seattle, which had done hundreds of transplants for a variety of diseases over the past decade, had agreed to accept him and to proceed with an allogeneic transplant, utilizing the marrow of Andrews's brother.

Dr. Desforges assured Father Greer that in his case the latest delays in his transplant date would have no deleterious effects; his protein count had not risen since he had begun taking the mild doses of prednisone and melphalan. Unlike Andrews, his myeloma was not resistant to the drugs.

Father Greer heard her words, but they did not register. His body seemed to be giving him a contrary second opinion. He had a persistent cough, and the pain in his chest and at the spot low in his back, where the myeloma had first manifested itself, seemed ever present and stronger. Although he had formerly disregarded Dr. Desforges's advice to take a regular dose of Motrin—not wanting to "get dependent on painkillers"—he now took the medication three times a day.

As he awaited the arrival of Father Paul Moritz, a seventy-two-year-old retired priest whom Father Greer had known since the mid-1970s, when they were both members of the archdiocesan Priest's

Council and whom he had immediately liked because of his easy good nature and sure administrative hand, Father Greer discovered that the yawning maw of parish work still wanted to swallow him. He had taken himself off the marriage and baptism schedules and talked about spending more time outside the rectory (he had always favored friends along the coast during the hot months, he was never shy to admit), but the calendar on his desk was no less densely scheduled.

Natick Common, a few blocks down East Central Street, had been transformed from a maze of random, beaten-down footpaths into a lush suburban park with a refurbished bandstand; and Father Greer was the cleric of choice to deliver the invocation at the dedication. A woman who had been a parish stalwart and for years a CCD teacher, could no longer be cared for by her daughter and was about to be released from the hospital after a stroke; a nursing home would have to be found for her. Two of his seminary class-mates were now patients at St. Patrick's Manor, a nursing home; he had to make time to visit them. The open house for the lower church was about to take place, but the floor mats still hadn't arrived, pieces of the new wallpaper were already coming loose from the walls, and a key light over the main altar still needed to be installed. A hauler was ready to tackle the removal of the tons of debris at the cemetery. The dimly lit, old, and terribly inefficient rectory kitchen was about to be remodeled. The organ in the upper church had been found to be in horrible disrepair. CCD teachers would have to be recruited and readied for the fall.

As usual in the life of a parish priest, there were few true triumphs, only small—and often transitory—achievements. A temporary sat-isfaction might have been gotten from the sight of the expanse of black plastic now covering a portion of Mr. Andrew Lane's property across from the church or simply from the silence of the site, once so bustling with heavy machinery and workers. Mr. Lane had hit a number of snags: from ground soaked for years with leaking fuel oil to a softening condominium market to, as Father Greer had learned through the Natick grapevine, serious financial problems. He had fought Mr. Lane for years, but now all he could say was, "Poor guy; probably overextended himself."

Inevitably, as Father Greer made his calls, those who knew about his illness had questions, and he, in a brisk though not unfriendly manner, had a stock response: "Hoping for four weeks in the hospital, two months of recuperation, and if everything goes right, I should be back by Easter." It was as if he were describing a hernia operation or a hip replacement. He then proceeded immediately to the business at hand.

When Janet Hamilton urged Father Greer to slow his pace, he claimed that he already had, but equally, that Father Moritz "doesn't know the details here. I don't want to leave him a mess."

Cardinal Law had called Father Greer, and the two of them had settled on the idea of an interim administrator. This would guarantee Father Greer the support of his parish when he returned and the option of staying in the residence he had known for the past four years. "More of a family atmosphere for you, Joe," the cardinal had said. The decision also made sense administratively: there was hardly a surfeit of qualified pastors waiting for a post. Father Moritz was willing to come out of retirement for a short-term assignment. Father Greer could ease back into church work at his own pace as he was completing his recovery.

Father Greer had been taken with the cardinal's pastoral compassion, and so he was surprised when he received a phone call from a courteous but assiduous young man in the archdiocesan finance office.

After exchanging pleasantries and Boston network talk (a prelude to many archdiocesan business conversations—in this case Father Greer had gone to Boston College with the young man's father) the young man informed Father Greer that St. Patrick's was one of ten churches randomly selected for an audit and that he would need two days, with the pastor present, to complete his work.

Initially Father Greer was angry. Then, quickly, amused.

"Here's what I'll do for you," he said to the young man. "I won't give you two days, but I'll give you two hours. I know you've got a job to do. I'll tell you right now that I have two bank accounts that you are never going to know about. I've got money stuffed away for the renovation of our kitchen that you are not going to see and the chancery is not going to hear about. I'm here to care for people, not dollars, and besides, I have a degree in accounting, which is a very dangerous thing for a priest who wants to get things done with the least amount of red tape. Okay?"

Late one afternoon, when he was in nearby Framingham, Father

Greer was finally able to cross off an item that had appeared too many times on his daily list. He swung by St. Patrick's Manor, a facility with a capacity of 292 residents staffed by the Carmelite Sisters for the Aged and Infirm. He found Father Michael Finnegan* in his room. Although it was a hot, muggy late-summer day, Father Finnegan shuffled about on his walker wearing a sweater and jacket zippered to his neck, a vague, vacant smile on his face. All his windows were closed; it was stifling in the room. Father Greer railed against the weather and the victorious opponents of the Red Sox and, surmising that Finnegan might understand the comedy of archdiocesan efficiency experts, dropped in the audit. Father Finnegan laughed. And kept on laughing. He began to babble incoherently.

Father Greer found Father John Morrissey,* the second member of the St. John's class of 1958 he had come to see, reading in the dayroom. It was another one-way conversation; Father Morrissey had suffered a stroke earlier in the year, after his mother had died. He contorted his face in an effort to speak, but the words would not come.

Father Greer drove back to the rectory in silence. He did not even bother to turn on the radio.

"How can you do it?" he asked rhetorically over dinner that evening. He was alone, covering the rectory. "How can a man stay depressed or sullen or angry with God when presented with such absurdity and such tragedy? Imagine asking a man who just had two smacks of pneumonia, has one foot inside that isolation room and cancer smoldering in his body, to sit for two days so the chancery can determine whether or not he's doing his job right—the holy job of managing money and property, of course. The job they asked him to take on. And then to see two guys who walked the same hallways I did, who were young and alert and ready to save the world, guys my age, in such condition. Finnegan and I used to play basketball together. Morrissey was my roommate one year; a serious type, kept pretty much to himself. Here was one man who wanted to talk, but couldn't; another who talked and had nothing to say.

"How can you take yourself seriously—feel sorry for yourself—after that? They aren't going to get that much better. I at least have a hope for a cure. How can Joe Greer hold on to his Black Irish, Jansenistic, semifatalist side? What's wrong with me?"

In early September rumors flew around St. Patrick's as parishioners saw less and less of their pastor. One had him already in the hospital, undergoing the transplant. Another, rejected for the transplant. Still another, that he would never be well enough to return to the parish. He had had holes drilled in his chest. He was days away from death.

Father Greer could have put an end to these rumors with a simple note in the Sunday bulletin, but he decided not to say anything until he was already in the hospital. He knew about parish rumors— during the busing crisis, there had been talk of marauding gangs of armed blacks from South Roxbury about to descend on St. Mark's in Dorchester, of white girls being molested by blacks at the integrated schools—and he knew that to respond to each preposterous story would be useless. With Father Moritz now in residence, living in one of the small guest rooms off the third-floor common room, Father Greer was frequently gone from the rectory. He returned few phone calls. Even close friends had difficulty reaching him.

As he had been a model in facing his disease and seeking treatment—never missing an appointment at New England Medical Center throughout the sometimes painful, often time-consuming pretransplant regimen—he tried "wasting time with God" as the day neared when he would be admitted to the hospital. His spiritual director, Father Joseph Payne, had prescribed doing less rather than more, and it took a new kind of discipline.

Father Greer's spiritual life had indeed changed since the Palm Sunday two years before when a searing pain in his back had heralded the onset of his disease. He claimed he was not as driven, was more meditative, more open—both to God and to people. His philosophy of "If it can't be taken care of in an hour, it can't be taken care of at all," his *modus operandi* of three decades in the priesthood that had stood him in such good stead for everything from counseling sessions to leaking gutters, had been abandoned.

During the previous two years, as Dr. Desforges had directed the quest for a bodily cure, Father Payne had monitored his spiritual well-being. An exemplary patient, Father Greer gave himself a more modest appraisal for his cooperation with the efforts of the Dominican prior. Dr. Desforges was working with a basically healthy man with a fatal disease, employing the latest in medical learning and technology; Father Payne, with a man of deep, if conventional, spirituality and an inner strength that had seen him through years of tumultuous changes in his church and in his own life.

Yet now, as he faced the reality of the months ahead, Father Greer sensed something was still lacking.

Father Payne had conducted literally hundreds of retreats over the years and counseled innumerable men and women religious. He knew the type of person he was dealing with. "The parish priest has an amazing number of contacts with people—but whom can he be truly intimate with?" he asked one afternoon as we sat and talked in the simple, institutionally furnished room at St. Stephen's Priory in Dover where he sees those who come to him for spiritual direction. Father Payne is a tall, bearded man with warm hazel eyes who rarely wears his white Dominican habit during his workday. His voice is low and reassuring. "There is a fraternity among diocesan priests, but it is often a surface closeness. And so these men, trained to work tirelessly and without muttering the slightest complaint, are relentlessly driven—by themselves. And when you combine that with the sense of insecurity they must feel about their role and their future in today's church, it's easy to see why they drive themselves so hard—both to prove they are worthwhile and to keep in constant motion, so the deep-seated anxieties can never surface. I gave a retreat in Providence to a group of diocesan priests, and each night they had to play Trivial Pursuit. They had trouble being alone and keeping silence.

"There is a real seduction in work as a parish priest, a false god, really, regardless of how much good the work does. One of the key barriers to wholeness and happiness as a religious today is the simple misunderstanding of an individual's psychology. We were all trained to look up to ideals, to saints, and to regard ourselves as pathetically wanting. There is an enormous amount of energy spent trying to be *that good*—and when a person fails, the guilt can be overwhelming. I like the quote from *The Little Black Child* by Blake, something to the effect that 'We are put on earth for a little space that we may learn to bear the beams of love.' That is what being a spiritual director is all about, focusing on the other person and seeing the unique light that shines upon them."

At the beginning of the summer, just about the time Father Greer had learned he was a candidate for a transplant, Father Payne had recommended that he read a book on the enneagram, an approach he often uses with his directees. The enneagram, of Sufi origin, is a method that helps the individual recognize the compulsions that developed early in life when he or she tried to become more acceptable to parents and other significant people and, once those compulsions are understood, to "convert" them into healthy mental and spiritual activity.

Father Greer, to whom Sufism—and, for all practical purposes, all Eastern spirituality—was so much "hocus-pocus," as he had often said, reluctantly began to read the book. It was more a testament to his affection for Father Payne than any sign of respect for his judgment on such things. But as he read, it was not difficult for him to see himself as a "number one" and "number three." There it was in print: "[ONES] are dedicated to being perfect and to doing things in a perfect way. . . . The compulsion of the THREE is to avoid failure. THREES grew up thinking their own personal worth consisted simply in the success of their achievements. . . . To them success includes efficiency. . . . Since the success of their enterprise is all important, they not only sacrifice their lives for it, but also expect others to be willing to make similar personal sacrifices . . . They do have strong personal feelings but these are put aside to be considered at some other time."

And while Father Greer never felt he fully understood the technique and never took time to participate in one of the weekend enneagram seminars the priory offered, the book stirred something inside him. It reaffirmed what the battery of psychological tests given him as a transplant candidate had said: he was practical, orderly, logical, realistic.

Both these tests and the enneagram drew Father Greer as an ideal Roman Catholic priest of his generation: directed, hard-working, dependable. And Father Payne was quick to underscore that these were valuable traits.

But compulsively exercised, they were also barriers to a life of faith and intimacy with God.

"With any real digging into yourself in spiritual direction," Father Payne pointed out to me, "the level of self-awareness is scary. What you find. What God calls on you to do. The person often feels it is better to just keep moving on."

Father Greer's usual approach was to confront a problem directly—be it a lapse in his own prayer life (set time aside and pray more) or the dingy lower church at St. Patrick's (raise the money and renovate it)—but as he faced a medical procedure that promised no long-term cure even if it did not kill him outright, he was left without any direct, logical path to follow.

"Joe Greer has always been the man in the driver's seat," Father Greer explained one night as he sat in his recliner, "and while I've made all this noise about giving up my will, about abandonment, I think I've talked a better game than I've played. Perfectionism and control. When I did my spiritual reading, it was a contest of how many pages I could turn. I would map out a beautiful twenty-five-minute prayer, a perfect thirty-minute meditation, and when nothing happened, I'd be dissatisfied, angry. My prayer life was not affective, and it wasn't effective. When plans didn't come through, I got boiling mad. Father Greer, the center of the universe; the world revolves around me.

"And after all, the whole transplant thing was calculated and precise, medical science; how could it be going to hell? 'Look, God, Joe Greer is doing it right. Why aren't you coming through on Your half of the bargain?' Those days and nights in Scotland began to sober me up. My depression was the result of centering on myself.

"And then the enneagram began to drum it into my thick skull: a man who has trouble accepting imperfection, who is a bug on neatness—if one of my priests leaves a cup, I'll pick it up; I can't resist!—who thinks wasting any time is a mortal sin, who won't let a person go on for more than the block of time I set—is this a man open to God's mercy? To God's voice? To His healing?

"It was painful to discover myself. To realize that I've said all the right things, but that the words haven't penetrated my being. That I was relentlessly demanding of others and myself. I've said all along that we learn from adversity, not success, and that this illness was the best teacher I ever had, but now I was being struck to the core. A core so hard and impenetrable I didn't want to touch it. I was slowly realizing that if the cancer was marching through my body, I wasn't in control anyhow. Joe Greer wasn't in the driver's seat anymore; he was in the rumble seat.

"My changeover came slowly, very slowly. Nothing dramatic."

Father Greer began to read a paragraph of Scripture instead of a chapter, a few lines from a book on spirituality instead of three pages. He put down the book. He daydreamed. He went for long walks on the bike trail at the Old Man of the Mountain near his ski house in New Hampshire. After his sessions with Father Payne, he walked by the pond at St. Stephen's Priory.

"And the simple discovery came: that God loves me not for what I do, but just because I exist. He loves me first; I don't have to earn that love. I went from words and actions to presence.

"I began not to judge so quickly. That if my priests weren't there for a meal, I didn't automatically think they were out socializing; they might have something more important to do. And I begin to feel a great peace.

"And something else: a premonition. Of loneliness.

"Although I felt God very much with me, I knew that I would be so alone during the transplant. I would be facing the great test of my life. I was facing death—which never frightened me—but also the *means* of death, which could be horrible. At once I was strong, and I knew I would be so weak very shortly. But I was ready, finally ready, for that room. The Lord would be with me there. In my pain, I could identify with His suffering. And I would be a better person—physically and spiritually—when I got out.

" 'Be not afraid.' It was always a favorite of mine. I finally understood those three simple words."

3

But we're like madmen stretching our hands to clasp the moon reflected in water.

The heavy mahogany table in the spacious first-floor dining room at St. Patrick's rectory is, like other places where seasoned professionals gather—say, a bar in a military club, safe but not far from a conflict, or a Formica counter in the coffee room just off a hospital's intensive care unit—a site close to tasks so difficult, daily, and grueling that they rarely can be discussed straightforwardly. In such places tragedy and triumph cannot be treated unambiguously and are instead cloaked in humor, the only acceptable guise.

In Catholic rectories, humor is an especially important ingredient these days. Not only has the once-admired profession of the priesthood been badly battered, but the work priests have always done still has to go on, with or without the approbation and automatic respect that once attended it. And humor does seem to reign in many places where priests gather. Sometimes it is forced, but more often not. It constitutes the acceptable currency of exchange among most priests, who for the most part are blessedly lacking in bitterness and acrimony. Most of the bitter ones have left, and those with acrid dispositions who have stayed, for whatever reason, usually limit to the strictly necessary the occasions at which they face themselves and their confreres.

It is not that the thousands of deaths and funerals at which the five men assembling around the St. Patrick's table have officiated or the human agonies they have witnessed have not left their collective mark on them or that they are immune to human suffering. Equally, it is not that they do not have stories to tell of towering bravery and faith. But to talk of agonies and heartbreaks—even those of the previous week, or since they last came together—can easily fill the midday half hour they have with each other and cast a pall over the time when they are supposed to put work aside and engage each other as men living in community. Besides, to talk of triumphs would be considered bragging or sanctimonious, jejune. Such tales would also be suspect, as successes are sparse and fleeting in the life of a parish priest.

In this dining room and ones like it across the country, the parish priest can enter a world that is comfortable for him. Parishioners, with their limited understanding of his life and their schizophrenic reverence/suspicion toward him, do not intrude here; only the clerical aristocracy—faded, less powerful, but still a sacred club, the royalest of the royal priesthoods offered in this earthly life.

It was meant to be this way. The priesthood was supposed to offer its exclusive membership, with amenities, services, and built-in companionship such that consecrated men would not seek the company of strangers. From golf and vacation partners to ready mealtime companions, comrades were always available. Ideally, priests living in common were to form a community much like the early Christians, their forebears in the priestly order, sharing their lives with one another.

And while most parish priests might not bond to each other easily, their life together is certainly more than that of a fraternal order: less than the ideal, more than the stereotype.

Mealtime at St. Patrick's—especially those rare meals like this one when all the priests are in attendance, none of them off on personal or parish business—is not a time for intimate personal sharing or deep theological discussion. Around this table, a priest can admit he is tired from being up all night with an accident victim, but he would never say it to court sympathy or praise. More likely he would tell of the separated parents he encountered, arguing over the comatose body of a son they both suddenly adore after years of marginal interest in his life, or the miserable coffee machine that demanded a second and third collection before delivering a cup of lukewarm water.

Father Greer, at the head of the table, standing before his bowl of Anna Caruso's fine minestrone soup (Father Moritz, Father Rossi, and Monsignor Mahoney were likewise having soup; Father Mullaney, who has a high cholesterol count, had a green salad and glass of white wine before him), was in his last week at St. Patrick's prior to the transplant. He was due to begin oral chemotherapy in two days and two days after that to be admitted to New England Medical Center.

"Bless us, O Lord, and these thy gifts, which we are about to receive from Thy bounty, through Christ Our Lord," he led the prayer that had not changed since they learned it as children.

"Amen," they responded in unison and sat.

The past weeks had indeed been eventful for Father Greer, but he retold the events to the men with whom he lives only in scant detail. Two weeks ago, under local anesthetic, he had had an eighteen-inch-long Hickman catheter, a silicone-and-plastic tube one sixteenth of an inch thick, implanted in the subclavian vein just under his collarbone. With the aid of a visiting nurse each morning he had learned, under sterile procedure, how to cleanse the site where the tube emerges from his chest and to flush, with a mild solution of the anticoagulant heparin in a hypodermic needle, the three color-coded lumens that branch off from the main tube. The catheter was not needed now but would be essential later, as he would be at risk of infection during the transplant. The catheter's Medusa-like array of lumens would allow blood, antibiotics, other drugs, and nutrition to be given intravenously for at least two months.

And within the past week, Father Greer had been party to a series of odd and, for him, remarkable incidents. While he had said little of those events to his fellow priests, they had had a profound effect upon him.

A charismatic prayer group at St. Joseph's, his old parish in Quincy, had invited him to their healing service, and although such emotional religiosity is hardly to his taste, he had gone. Father Greer, a priest who had anointed so many of the sick, had been urged by these laypeople to allow himself to be anointed with oil by them. He had felt uneasy with the request. In his mind, he had gone through a quick checklist of the canonical propriety of such an act, and while he had not been sure of either its efficacy or its seemliness, he had allowed his forehead, lips, ears, and hands to be blessed. He had been prayed over, first in words he could discern, then in tongues, an eerie, high-pitched cry to heaven for his well-being. As he had given his blessing, a woman had swooned, then passed out. She had been gently helped to a comfortable position on the floor and had been left there as the service continued.

A drug addict who had come to see Father Greer at the rectory for counseling had asked for some holy water, which she hoped would help her in times of temptation. When she had heard from Father Greer the reason he could not see her the next week, she had thrust her hand, dripping with the holy water, across the desk and onto his forehead, where she had made a sign of the cross. He had again been taken aback but had not resisted.

One parishioner had brought him water from the shrine at Lourdes, another a medal from Medjugorje, Yugoslavia, both sites venerated by Catholics because the Blessed Virgin is reported to have appeared there. (The second parishioner had wanted a picture of Father Greer to take to Medjugorje, but he had declined this request.) He had been given scapulars, a Miraculous Medal, and other medals, including that of St. Peregrine, the patron saint of cancer victims. (According to tradition, the fourteenth-century saint, as an act of penance, stood whenever it was not necessary to sit, and this was thought to have caused a cancerous sore to develop on his leg. A surgeon said the leg would have to be amputated. The night before the operation was to be performed, St. Peregrine prayed before an image of the crucified Christ, and the next morning the sore was found to be healed.)

The events were certainly happenstance and spontaneous, but in his relatively uniform—and unlikely—responses, Father Greer felt he had made a small breakthrough. He had allowed people the opportunity to help in his cure.

Just as he had served them, he was trying to let them minister to him. Each was an isolated and short episode; he was not about to change a lifetime of reserve and throw himself and his illness before them, but he wanted people somehow to come away with the thought "He needs us now, too."

Also, within these past days Father Greer had begun to be more successful at "wasting time with God," as Father Payne had urged him to. With this relaxation of his normally disciplined approach to spirituality, his conscious meditation and random thoughts had coalesced. The transplant and the attendant solitude would provide a unique opportunity to offer up his suffering, his burnt oblation to God. He would approach the transplant with faith, leaving its outcome in God's hands. During his recovery, he would practice the discipline called "centering prayer," in which mantralike repetitions of words ("Father," "Heaven," "Lord") or short phrases ("Lord, have mercy," "Come, Lord Jesus") clear the mind and promote a new awareness.

He was positive, almost upbeat, about the procedure. In the physical realm, he saw it as a chance to gain years of life, or—if he was one of the unfortunate 20 percent of transplant patients who could not regenerate blood cells or who had other serious complications from the chemotherapy or radiation—to meet with a quick and honorable death. Spiritually, even given the dangers he sensed he would face in room 664, his bone marrow transplant presented an opportunity for another kind of rebirth.

And so with all these cosmic issues churning about in Father Greer's life, the conversation around the dining room table at St. Patrick's on this day in September began with . . .

"Bedding." Father Greer pronounced the word with a deadpan look on his face.

"Musty. Tattered. We needed some new bedding up in New Hampshire, so Billie [Father William] O'Connor—who reads the newspaper ads like they were Sacred Scripture—and I go into this discount house where Billie said they had a great sale. Pretty junky stuff, so we drive over to Filene's, where they are also having a sale, and these seem better. A good buy, so Billie tells me. I ask the saleslady to get us four pillows, four bedspreads, and some sheets. She's about to put all this together when who comes along but Betty Jensen, you know, the head of our Altar Society, and she asks us what we're doing. 'Bedding, Mrs. Jensen.' She looks a little perturbed. Turns out she's a supervisor over there, gets a whopping employee discount off everything, and we never asked. The price keeps going down. Bingo, we save sixty bucks and she's dropping them by the rectory. Don't even have to lug them out of the store. Ah, the power of the collar."

Father Moritz weighed in with his story of clerical privilege—a winter vacation to Hawaii on someone else's frequent flier bonus—and then Father Greer continued. "Sometimes the collar helps, and sometimes it strangles you," he said. "The other day, I was in getting some skivvies and T-shirts to send over to Jim Canniff's for when I get out of the hospital and there's this long line, so I stand in it like everybody else. Oh, no. 'Come right ahead, Father,' the checkout lady says, and the waters part and I'm up in front. 'We give a clerical discount,' she says proudly, and when she tries to crank that into this fancy computer that passes for a cash register, the thing goes nuts. Buzzing. Lights flashing. 'Don't worry, Father, we can work this out.' I smile kind of weakly at the people in line, but they aren't smiling. All for a buck-forty. How many churchgoers did I lose with that one?"

The cheese was passed, and the latest archdiocesan clergy moves were gone over in short order and shorthand—"Got fed up at charities; said he wanted out." "Cancer, wasn't it, for Monk? Didn't last six months." "Henry had a bit of a drinking problem, I hear; who wouldn't at that place?" "The grade school was killing Mike, and he said to the personnel board, 'Transfer me or I'll transfer myself' "—before the conversation spun back to clerical privilege, or the lack of it, for nuns. "A shame," Father Rossi said about the present. "People still think they're lilies of the field and don't need anything." Then he jumped back decades to the behind-the-scenes power of the legendary German nun Sister Pasqualina, known as "la Popessa," supposedly the true power behind Pope Pius XII. "You wanted to see him, you saw her first," Father Mullaney said.

"Reminds me of a pope joke," said Father Moritz over tea. "There's one of those huge outdoor papal audiences in St. Peter's Square and the crowd is screaming, 'Papa, Papa,' so enraptured to see their pope standing, right there, on the balcony. Then one of the cardinals comes out to announce that the pope is dying. Rosaries come out, signs of the cross, everybody kneels down and there's a lot of buzzing. Prayers being said. 'Papa, papa,' they say reverently. The cardinal tells them that only a kidney transplant will save their beloved leader. He brings out a white feather and sends it off, floating over the crowd, and tells them whoever it lands on will be privileged to donate a kidney. 'Papa, papa,' " Father

Moritz mimicked the faithful in attendance, but this time the P's had sufficient plosion to blow the feather away. The priests smiled broadly.

"Last clerical privilege story," said Father Greer, rolling his napkin and stuffing it into a holder. "I know the golf pro at this fancy country club—Bretton Woods, in Mount Washington, New Hampshire—so four of us stop there on the way back from the chalet one afternoon. And just as we arrive, there walking up to the first tee are a threesome of very nice Jewish ladies. The starter waves us through: 'Go, ahead, Fathers.' 'I thought it was ladies first,' one of the ladies says. I'm about to agree with her when the starter whispers to them. 'Men of the cloth,' he says reverently, as if we were on the most urgent of sacred missions. 'Men of the cloth.' Jewish-Christian relations, go back two steps."

In this, his last week at St. Patrick's, Father Greer decided to say a daily private Mass in his room, which he did at about six o'clock, at a table by the window overlooking East Central Street. With the delays in his transplant date and the number of rumors floating around the parish, Father Greer found too many of his parishioners giving him what he called a "grave look" every time they saw him. Eventually it became too emotional for him.

"They were trying to bury me," he said. "Who were they looking at when they saw me? I've seen people with cancer, and I didn't look like that. I feel pretty good. Do I look like a man with cancer? But maybe they were doing what I'm doing: counting the days. 'This is my last Monday, my last Tuesday.' The end of my mortal life may be just five days away now. It's tough on people, too; especially after my homily on Sunday, which most knew would be my last. For a while, anyhow.

"Using the scripture about it not being good for man to be alone, I talked about dependence and how, when we were kids, we were so dependent on God and then we lost it as adults. We got independent; I told them I was independent and proud and thought I could do anything I set my mind to. I learned I didn't have all the control I thought I did in my life. Actually, that I had very little and that I was learning to depend on God more. I pointed up to the crucifix: the horizontal beam is the relationship with our fellow man; the vertical, our dependency on God. That was the cross we took up every day, and if we avoided that, we were avoiding people and we were turning our backs on God. We were telling him we could do just fine without Him. I didn't really mention my illness, but they knew what was behind it all and there were some pretty long faces when I greeted people after the Mass. Just too emotional. I wanted to slip away quietly.

"But I surprised myself at the end of the homily. There they were, words coming out of my mouth. 'I love you. I'll miss you.'

"I've thought about weakness a lot this week. And about God's love. And how He loves us first because we are His and nothing we can do will ever destroy that love. Funny, I never thought about my transgressions, the times I sinned, the worst times. I think that's a temptation anyhow, and especially at a time like this. Not to accept a person's own weakness, not to accept God's forgiveness."

We were talking in the living room, Father Greer sitting in his customary place on the lounge chair. What he was talking about went to the roots of his soul, but his tone of voice was little different from that I had heard in our first meeting over a year before.

On Father Greer's desk in the next room was a huge bottle of capsules and a smaller bottle. They rested on the corner of the desk calendar, the month of October. The month was blank. Only the faint indentations from previous commitments and appointments indicated that this was out of the ordinary. The capsules in the larger bottle each contained ninety milligrams of melphalan, the anticancer drug he had taken before. In the smaller bottle were ten-milligram tablets of Compazine, an antinausea medication. Beginning the next morning and for each of the three following days, Father Greer was supposed to take forty-five melphalan capsules, getting them down in whatever combinations he could. The maximum dose he had previously taken had been eight a day. When Father Greer had left the prescription for the melphalan at a local drugstore, the pharmacist had called Dr. Shulman to make sure the dosage was correct. He had never filled a prescription of the drug directing such massive doses.

The pharmacist's call had given Dr. Shulman a reason to do something she had been hoping she would have a chance to do: phone Father Greer at the rectory. Up to that point she had hesitated, but felt their relationship had gotten stronger since she had seen him through his pneumonia, and she badly wanted him to know that her concern for him was not limited to the times she had seen him in the hematology/oncology clinic. She knew from experience that patients feel closer to their doctor after an illness; the doctor has "pulled them through," whether he or she played any significant role or not. Actually Dr. Shulman had had very little to do for Father Greer during his second hospitalization for pneumonia.

She was also aware of how she presented herself. As a brilliant chemistry and physics major at Harvard, she had often heard from her classmates that she was too intense, too driven. She had begun to loosen up with Father Greer and had even begun to joke with him at the clinic. He had proved to be a willing partner: on the last visit he had asked her if she was Italian, as she "talked with her hands."

"Even though I've read everything about this transplant and what's going to happen to me, it's funny that it ends up being so vague, so unbelievable in my mind," Father Greer said that evening after supper as we sat in his suite. "Whatever it is, I don't want it to be a cross; I want it to be a stepping-stone. But that's so much intellectualizing. I know it's out of my hands now. The man who was always serving people and was so independent will soon be totally dependent on people. Or in five days I could be dead. Or at best, nausea, depression, loneliness.

"What I wonder most of all is what I'll be like when I get back. Will I be fit to be a pastor again? Will I have the stamina? Will I have all my marbles? There certainly is a sadness right now, but I haven't cried, no," he said in response to my question. "My training was not to show my emotions. My pride won't let me cry. But the tears are right there," he said, pointing behind his eyes, his voice now thicker. "After all, this parish is my family, and I'm going to be leaving them soon."

As he had been told to do, Father Greer began the melphalan the next day, a Wednesday, managing to ingest thirty-five pills. He also took the maximum Compazine dosage. The following day he could take only a dozen melphalans, his nausea was so intense. He called Dr. Desforges and said he could not take any more of the pills because he would throw up. Again. She told him to try to stick it out one more day and if he could not tolerate the medication to come in to the hospital the next morning and be admitted.

Father Greer had planned to see Father Payne on Friday, his last day before he was scheduled to be admitted, and receive from him the Sacrament of the Sick. By Friday morning he knew that would be impossible; he had to get to the hospital. He called Dan Barry, a parishioner who is an undertaker and usually available. Barry appeared at the church office within minutes.

His bags already in the car, Father Greer told Janet Hamilton to keep an eye on the cemetery excavation, to call town hall if the payment was not received soon for the parking lot lease, and to keep after the contractors who were to renovate the kitchen. He stood in the office, his eyes more bloodshot than usual and somewhat glassy, wondering if he had left any detail unsettled.

When he stopped talking, there was silence.

"Don't worry, Father," Janet said, her eyes filling with tears. "We'll do our best."

"I'll see you in a month," he said to Janet, to Ann Garvey, who had just happened by, and to Father Moritz, the only priest in the rectory at the time (Father Rossi was out on Communion calls, and Father Mullaney was presiding at a funeral). "I hope." Janet and Ann hugged him and Father Moritz shook his hand.

"As they say in the Good Book, my time has come," Father Greer said, and walked out of the office.

On Janet's desk, Father Greer had left a handwritten note that was to appear in the St. Patrick's bulletin that Sunday under the heading "From the Pastor's Desk."

" 'Father, how are you feeling? When are you going to the hospital?' I am feeling great and I am now in the hospital. On Saturday, October 8th, I was admitted to the New England Medical Center, the Proger Building. I am in the Bone Marrow Transplant Room, an isolation room. (No visitors, no flowers.) At the present time I am having total body irradiation as well as chemotherapy; it is thru this treatment that the multiple myeloma will be eliminated in my bone marrow. After the multiple myeloma is eliminated, the bone marrow taken from my body in July will be infused into my body once again and hopefully will start to grow. I will remain in this room for a period of four to six weeks in order that my bone marrow may grow in a bacteria-free environment.

"After the first step, I will leave the hospital and stay in a rectory near the hospital in sanitized rooms for a couple of months. During this time I will be on a special diet, receiving blood transfusions and antibiotics to fight infection. When my marrow is once again healthy and my white cells back to their proper level, we will have won the battle.

"So it seems that if everything goes according to schedule, I will see you sometime in the early part of next year—I will try to keep you informed as to how my recovery is going and at this time let me wish you and your families all the best for the coming holiday season and I ask you occasionally to remember me in your prayers.

God Bless,
Father Greer

4

*Now what's wrong? What on earth's the matter? I hadn't
realized there were tears on my face, I wasn't even thinking
of it.*

The procedure that could save Father Greer's life was itself a by-
product of one of the world's most powerful instruments of calculated death. It was only after the detonation of the atom bombs at
Hiroshima and Nagasaki that medical science began to comprehend
the power of massive doses of radiation. And only after those days
of death did the U.S. Atomic Energy Commission (AEC)—realizing that not only innocent civilians but, in the future, combat
troops could be at risk—begin research into what might be done
for victims of radiation poisoning.

So, the history of bone marrow transplants is a short one. Dr.
Edwin Osgood at the University of Oregon Medical School was
perhaps the first to attempt to infuse marrow. In 1938 and 1939
Osgood and his medical team in Portland gave donor marrow to
three patients with aplastic anemia, a disease in which marrow stops
producing blood cells. All three suffered excruciating deaths in
which their skin erupted and organs such as the kidneys and liver,
which had been functioning normally before the procedure, shut
down. Osgood initially concluded that bone marrow transplants,
while theoretically beneficial, had no value for his patients and that
he had both shortened their lives and visited horrible suffering upon
their last days.

When thousands of Japanese continued to die weeks after the

atomic bombs' explosion in August 1945, many as a result of aplastic anemia, it was clear that radiation was responsible for their deaths, damaging their marrow and preventing it from generating the blood cells necessary to sustain life. Research began under the auspices of the AEC to investigate how living creatures could be shielded from this radiation and what could be done when such exposure occurred. After an extended battle with the military establishment, President Harry Truman put this research arm under civilian control, and the results of the AEC experiments, which could have ended up as classified documents, were made available to the medical research community.

Around 1950, Dr. L. O. Jacobson at the University of Chicago, working under an AEC grant, found that mice subjected to lethal amounts of radiation could be saved by shielding their spleens. He made the crucial connection: new blood cells were not some randomly produced entity, and those housed in the spleen could repopulate the body. These cells, eventually called hematopoietic stem cells, might, Jacobson deduced—although he could not see or identify them—be able to repopulate the blood if injected into a mouse after a lethal dose of radiation. Mice were blasted with X rays, then infused with marrow containing stem cells taken from other mice, and they lived—at least for a while. Eventually they developed symptoms similar to those of Osgood's patients, and it was finally discovered that the marrow graft was actually attacking the host body. The marrow seemed to sense it was in hostile territory and generated antibodies to defend itself; the host, its immune system suppressed by the radiation, could not resist. Thus, graft-versus-host disease was inadvertently discovered.

In the 1950s and 1960s, bone marrow transplants in humans were done more or less randomly as a treatment of last resort when there was no other hope for the patient. Transplants were occasioned by chance, not choice, as in an atomic reactor accident in Yugoslavia where five men were exposed to lethal levels of radiation. Four survived after a marrow transplant, but physicians had no idea if it was their action that had saved the men; they could not repeat the procedure under similar conditions, which is the key to truly useful research. Eventually, mice—this time from an inbred colony developed by the Nobel laureate George Snell—and then the inbred

beagles of E. Donnell Thomas provided genetically similar experimental subjects, so that transplant experiments could be duplicated.
It turned out that *sibling* marrow was effective among lower animals.
And so when Thomas went to Pittsburgh in 1967 to transplant the
marrow of a man who had been exposed to 600 rads of radiation
in an industrial accident, using the marrow of his identical twin,
he had an ideal opportunity to prove his theory. Not only did the
transplant take, but the recipient outlived his brother, who later
died of a heart attack.

Thomas moved to the Fred Hutchinson Cancer Center in Seattle,
which was to become the most active transplant center in the world,
and began work on leukemia patients, killing their marrow with
drugs and radiation and then rescuing them with genetically
matched marrow. His early work yielded depressing results. Graft-
versus-host disease and other side effects caused the death of 90
percent of his patients, leading researchers in other centers to pro-
nounce the procedure not worth the risks. But that 10 percent—
people with aplastic anemia and acute leukemia, diseases that
inevitably would have proved fatal, some of whom are still alive
today—made up the Seattle center's counterargument.

Transplant centers sprang up around the country in the 1970s—
one of them at the New England Medical Center—but most quickly
closed. Patients were dying, many of them experiencing deaths more
horrible than their disease alone would have accorded them, and
the drain on physicians and nurses and the families of patients was
more than most hospitals wanted to bear.

But at Seattle, at UCLA, and at a hospital in Villejuif, France,
transplants continued. With them came an increased understanding
of the optimum dosage of powerful drugs and radiation that would
kill cells and not the patient, the best time in a patient's illness to
intercede, how much marrow to reinfuse, and, just as important,
the period of time in which that marrow should be given. Patient
management issues, such as isolation rooms to reduce infections,
were painstakingly and painfully discovered. Better antibiotics were
utilized. Blood banking, the necessary interim step, was perfected
so that patients would not die from complications of improperly
matched transfusions.

By 1979, not only were allogeneic transplants, where the marrow came from a genetically matched donor, being performed, but autologous transplants as well, with the patient's own marrow being returned to his or her own body. Finally, by the early 1980s, bone marrow transplants were the treatment of choice for certain cancers and blood diseases such as acute myeloid leukemia and acute lymphoblastic leukemia. Eighty percent of aplastic anemia patients could now be saved; before the transplants were developed, all of them would have died. Half the patients with Hodgkin's disease who were resistent to chemotherapy were cured or had long remissions, as well as 30 to 50 percent of all those with leukemia. Follow-up time, posttransplant, extended past ten years for some.

While autologous transplants were theoretically more desirable because recovery time was shortened and graft-versus-host disease was eliminated, researchers knew that the marrow they were reinfusing probably contained—though greatly diminished by the drugs and radiation—small numbers of cancerous cells that could eventually reinfect the patient. And so peripheral stem cells began to receive new attention. If these immature cells, which were thought to be disease-free, could be extracted from the bloodstream and returned to germinate in the bone marrow, the patient's body in essence would be returned to its predisease state.

While the acute and chronic leukemias, Hodgkin's disease, lymphomas, and aplastic anemia received primary attention—being diseases that attacked bodies young enough to withstand the assault of radical treatment—multiple myeloma was relegated to medical science's back burner, as it usually struck the old.

When Drs. Jane Desforges and Kenneth Miller had proposed reopening the transplant unit at New England Medical Center two years earlier, in 1986, they were building on the competence of other transplant centers which, in a short period of time, had developed successful treatment methods. Of the 9,500 transplants done in ninety centers worldwide, most had been done in the two years previous. It was a young field, growing in experience and producing encouraging survival rates. But Desforges and Miller also wanted to attack the unattackable: multiple myeloma. At the time of the unit's opening on Proger 6 North, they considered three of their myeloma patients strong transplant candidates: Father Greer, John Andrews, and Joe Johnson. They wanted to do more for these men than prescribe increasingly larger doses of drugs, to which the mye-loma patients' bodies would eventually become resistant. They wanted to try to save these lives, not just extend them for a few months or years.

Dr. Jane Desforges is a world-renowned hematologist, the author or coauthor of nearly two hundred medical journal articles and chapters in medical texts, an associate editor of one of the most prestigious medical publications, *The New England Journal of Medicine*, and, since 1973, the senior hematologist at the New England Medical Center. While her research has certainly been recognized, Dr. Desforges is best known within the hematology world as an expert clinician. She is a doctor who never seems harried, who answers even the simplest question from a patient fully and with patience. She is often chosen the best teacher of the year at Tufts School of Medicine, though residents and interns can find her quite demanding and impatient at their lapses in knowledge, especially when their assessment of cases obfuscates rather than illuminates. She is sixty-seven years old, forty-three years a doctor; during that time she has trained scores of young hematologists.

One of them, Dr. Miller, who is forty-two, after his residency at New York University, fellowship at New England Medical Center, and visits to the leading transplant centers in Boston and New York, started the New England Medical Center's transplant unit, a pres-tigious assignment for so young a physician. He is an intense, balding man given to fidgeting in his chair when, rarely, he is seated. He speaks in short, choppy sentences, runs instead of walks, and exudes an air of impatience. He does not resemble Dr. Desforges's open, even parental, presence. Some would call him cold.

They work together at one of the leading hematology centers in the world at a time when the specialty is experiencing explosive growth in research and treatment. Because of recent discoveries of the basics of blood production—such as why cells travel where they do in the body and new understanding of the biology of hematology, which promises the possibility of altering cells and not simply erad-icating them—many in medicine consider this a golden age of hematology.

Father Greer could not have been in better hands, or at a better place.

. . .

On Friday, October 7, the day before Father Greer was scheduled to be admitted, I visited the medical center to talk with the two doctors about their patient and his course of treatment.

"In the week ahead, we will use what is considered a method on the cutting edge of biotechnology," Dr. Desforges began. "Yet a few years from now we might look back and find this frightfully outdated. But we do not have the luxury of waiting; Father Greer will never be in a better condition, and if we don't move now, if we don't intervene, the myeloma will spread and he will surely die. It is not a desperation move, not at all. It is opportune; it is time.

"Because of the rapid advances in hematology, I have to admit I am continually a novice in the field." As she spoke, Dr. Desforges's warm smile took off, if not forty-three, at least twenty-three years. "That's encouraging. It's very humbling to have to say 'I don't know' or 'I'm not sure,' but we don't know some of the simplest facts— exactly why cells become cancerous and grow so rapidly, for instance. We are not sure we are giving the *right* treatment to Father Greer, but it certainly is the *best* that medical science can offer today. One of our major problems is that we are not very good at giving selective chemotherapy that just wipes out the myeloma cells, and we can't do much better than the blanket treatment of total body irradiation, because we just don't know where all the myeloma cells are. We are using a cannon to kill a fly."

They explained that the procedure Father Greer was to undergo was new not only in their center but throughout the world. There were perhaps ninety people with multiple myeloma who had been transplanted, most of them with allogeneic marrow transplants and most within the past few years. And while a handful had survived up to seven years posttransplant, the numbers of successful transplants and the follow-up time provided insufficient documentation that the treatment, rather than good fortune, was the cause.

The New England Medical Center unit had done some twenty-four transplants for other blood diseases and cancers, namely acute lymphocytic leukemia, Hodgkin's disease, and lymphoma, and their success rate, with 70 percent of their patients alive one year posttransplant, compared favorably with that of other, established transplant units in Boston hospitals, such as those at Dana-Farber, Brigham's and Women's, and Beth Israel. Father Greer would be the center's first transplant for multiple myeloma.

"His marrow is contaminated; we know that," Dr. Desforges continued. "We hope the stem cells we have extracted and the lymphocytic solution in which they are suspended are free of the disease. But after transplant, if a patient is not capable of regenerating the necessary white and red blood cells and platelets, plus the other blood components, we then can use the marrow we previously extracted. In that case, while the patient may do better for a while because we have reduced the severity of the disease, we will have failed.

"We want all our transplant patients well aware of the experimental nature of the procedure and the downside risks. We tell them all very explicitly what will happen to them, but every one of them will say afterwards, 'You told me, but I didn't know how bad it would be.' "

"We see very sick patients, and many of them die," Dr. Miller said, his words coming at a much more rapid pace than Dr. Desforges's. "It takes an enormous toll on you, seeing somebody slip away, having to tell the family there is no hope. But I think what attracts physicians to a field like this—at least in my case—is that if you are very good at what you do, you can make an enormous difference. And it is a clinical field at a time in medicine when many other specialties rely on the numbers, the tests. You have to listen to figure out what is really going on. The odds are against you all the time, but the prospects of effecting a cure, or of significantly extending a useful life, are what drives all of us on. And the future of transplants is boundless. What if we could isolate, cultivate, and preserve stem cells? The prospects of ridding people of disease are staggering, just staggering.

"I would say we are not of the 'death with dignity' school here. We don't want our patients to die and we fight with them every step of the way, and so it is the kind of work you don't forget about when you go home or on vacation or on a weekend off. You constantly ask yourself if you have covered all the bases. 'What am I not seeing?' 'Is there a better way?' "

To both of them Father Greer was the ideal patient. Physiologically, he was a robust man of thirty-five. Mentally, he was hopeful about a cure yet seemed ready to accept the consequences of a failure. This type of patient, they said, was the easiest to treat. "But there is another dimension, something quite different about him, that we don't often see; I think we both agree about that," Dr. Miller said, turning to his senior colleague.

"I sense it is faith," Dr. Desforges said. "That everything doesn't end with death. But it is neither a blind faith in physicians nor a blind faith that God will take care of it all. Other patients shy away from death; he doesn't. He is going into that isolation room with strength of a magnitude that we've not experienced before."

"The average patient looks to the physician for strength," said Dr. Miller. "And we encourage them to express their feelings, whatever they might be. Father Greer has not done that. As patients get sicker, they tend to bond to the doctor. But with Father Greer, the distance between patient and doctor hasn't changed, really, from when he first came in. There has been no transference. He has never truly confided in us, gotten angry, emotional. In a way, we wish he had. Because as he finds that he is no longer in control, it's much easier to have someone there you can turn to. Perhaps he is closer to Rebecca Shulman in a way. There he can be paternal. He is a man used to that role, used to being of service to others."

"Doctors will employ such a simple device as silence to bring out the patient," Dr. Desforges said. "We have given Father Greer many opportunities to come forth. But unlike most patients who, if you don't talk, they usually do, he is a man, obviously because of his training and discipline, not uncomfortable with silence."

"In a strange way, perhaps because of that unspoken quality of faith he has, he's treating us," Dr. Miller remarked. "He somehow wants to make it easy on us; he doesn't want to overburden us with concerns about him."

As we finished our conversation, I volunteered what I knew about Father Greer's difficulty taking the melphalan—I had last spoken to him the night before, on Thursday—and asked if he was tolerating the medication any better today. "You can find out yourself," Dr. Desforges said. "He's down in the clinic. We're admitting him a day early to help him through it."

I found him in the hematology/oncology clinic, seated next to a woman wearing an off-center wig of an unnatural brown color. Dan Barry had brought him to the hospital a half hour before and left. Across the expanse of rose carpeting were those faces with which Father Greer was now so familiar—faces with pale skin, glazed eyes, slightly parted lips. Father Greer had his glasses on and was looking down at a book, but it was obvious he was not reading.

Soon he was taken into one of the examining rooms and given an injection of Trilafon for his nausea. He was also given Benadryl as a sedative since the antinausea medication can cause the rigors— shaking and chills. Within minutes his stomach calmed. He then went to another building to have an electrocardiogram and X rays. These are part of standard admitting procedure. The X-ray machine was broken, and he had to wait almost an hour. As he waited he mentioned missing his appointment with Father Payne and also failing to get a haircut. "I guess I won't be needing it," he said about the haircut, forcing a smile.

Terry Fogaran was in the clinic when Father Greer returned and told him that the room on Proger 6 North to which he would be admitted—he was to enter the isolation room the following day— was not ready. "Would you like to go out for a bite to eat, Father? Feel well enough? Did they give you enough medicine for the nausea? Don't be a John Wayne about it."

"I feel more like Paulette Goddard," he replied.

"Was it a good week except for us spoiling it with the pills?" she asked, taking his arm.

"Yeah. Saw a woman with myeloma on Monday. Wednesday she was dead."

"Oh."

"So I'll go get a sandwich and a beer. The feast before the famine."

"Watch the beer; your count is down."

"Right, right."

We walked a few hundred feet to the Beer and Ale, a restaurant tucked into the ground floor of one of the New England Medical Center buildings. His pace was slow and he was not inclined to engage in casual conversation. Father Greer ordered a tuna salad and soon commented on the good taste of the cottage cheese that accompanied it, noting he hadn't had any solid food in three days. He sipped on iced tea.

At one o'clock he was formally admitted and told to go to Proger 6 North. He headed to the sixth floor, taking along his personal effects: a small suitcase, a cardboard box of religious videotapes, a quart bottle of Paul Masson Rosé, and a square leather case, his Mass kit. A nurse went through the floor's intake form, interjecting that she was from California, had worked at hospitals across the country, and had just started at the medical center.

"Why are you here?"

Father Greer answered the questions in a quiet, calm voice as he sat on the edge of his bed.

"What are your roles and responsibilities at home?"

"I'm a pastor."

"A pastor, yes?"

"Of eight thousand five hundred people."

"How has the illness affected your life?"

"I get tired easily. And I take things in proper perspective."

"Do you anticipate any problems in this hospital stay?"

Father Greer only smiled in response.

"I know. I know," she said softly.

The intake completed, Father Greer changed into a hospital nightshirt and crawled into bed. Within ten minutes he was fast asleep. He had not slept well the night before, and the Benadryl had induced an early-afternoon nap.

5

*First I was no more than a spark, an atom of the glowing
dust of divine charity. I am that again, and nothing more,
lost in unfathomable night. But now the dust-spark has
almost ceased to glow, it is nearly extinguished.*

Father Greer smiled at the sound of the word.

"Ablation. *Abstuli, ablatus.* 'To remove, dissipate.' Nice, tidy
way of putting it, no?"

Sue Tegan, although a Catholic, was one of a more recent vintage, and her parochial school education had left her innocent of
Latin. Tegan, the primary nurse assigned him for the duration of
his stay, returned the smile—though a bit quizzically—as she hung
the second bottle of clear liquid on the IV pole attached to his bed.
She inserted needles into two of the lumens on Father Greer's
catheter, which dangled from his chest.

The ablation—a "full-scale ablation" in proper medical terminology—of Father Greer's bone marrow began about the time St.
Patrick's parishioners were filing in for eight o'clock Sunday Mass
and reading his letter in the bulletin. Tegan first started a saline
solution, then opened the slide clamp for a bottle containing the
drug Cytoxan. Greek and Latin roots form the etymology of this
staple of chemotherapy: *cyto* for cell and *toxicum* for poison. Cell
poison.

The saline solution was set to pass through Father Greer's body
at a rate of one liter an hour, the Cytoxan at a steady drip that,
unless complications arose, would take about forty-five minutes.
The dosage of Cytoxan, five grams, was some ten to twenty times

what normal cancer patients might receive. The rate of the saline solution turned out to be as crucial as that of the Cytoxan since if Father Greer's bladder were not continuously filled and emptied as the "cell poison" passed through, a severe bladder inflammation or internal bleeding could result. Diluted in the saline solution were doses of Trilafon for nausea, as well as Ativan and Benadryl to mildly sedate him and alleviate anxiety. A Foley catheter had been inserted to purge his body of this toxic solution.

Cytoxan is still another of medicine's unexpected returns from the devastation of war. Mustard gas introduced into the arsenal of weapons in World War I inflicted burns, blindness, and death by destroying external and internal cells. In the postwar years the "prepared mind" of scientists—in this case in Germany, which had once used the nitrogen compound with awful effectiveness—sought a way to harness its lethal power. As the mustard gases caused low white blood cell counts, a logical jump was made to employ them in treating diseases in which the white cells ran rampant. At first, small doses of actual mustard gas were used on desperately ill cancer patients to help shrink their tumors. Many died from the treatment, but autopsies revealed that the tumor mass had been reduced. Further research eventually developed a family of alkylating agents with more limited side effects, which have been standard in cancer treatment for the past thirty years. While the specific action of Cytoxan is unknown, it somehow interferes with the growth of fast-dividing cells, perhaps skewing the DNA message as these cells divide. These defective cells can no longer reproduce and are rejected by the body, eventually to die and be sloughed off. As cancer cells—myeloma among them—divide the most rapidly, they readily fall victim to Cytoxan's toxic power. But the cannon, to use Dr. Desforges's analogy, also destroys both before and after it has hit its target. Healthy cells in every part of the body are in the line of fire. The cells in hair follicles and the gastrointestinal tract from mouth to anus, as well as those within the bone marrow, are also rapidly dividing cells, and they are equally decimated. After such massive doses of Cytoxan, the patient has a thin line across each fingernail, much like a tree ring, marking the days when normal cell growth was preempted.

Although the chemical action of Cytoxan does not disrupt the acid balance in the stomach for hours, the brain senses that a poison is being admitted and often sends a signal ordering its rejection. Halfway through the bottle of Cytoxan, Father Greer felt a wave of nausea but said nothing to Tegan. The drug continued to flow into his body. He did complain that his "taste buds are on neutral" and that he had an awful taste in his mouth.

That afternoon, despite being mildly fatigued after a poor night's sleep, he had had enough energy to ride more than two miles on the exercise bike in his room and to watch several hours of a videotape series on Catholicism by Father Richard P. McBrien. It amused him that while McBrien, who was a star student at Father Greer's own seminary, was now the head of Notre Dame University's theology department, he was, as Father Greer put it, "Banned in Boston" because of his liberal views. McBrien's popular syndicated column had been dropped from the archdiocesan paper, *The Pilot*.

On Monday morning Father Greer received the second Cytoxan treatment. He tolerated it equally well, although waves of nausea swept over him that afternoon. He rode another two miles on the bike and did not vomit. At supper he was able to manage only a little Jell-O and clear soup, his normally healthy appetite having abandoned him, but otherwise he felt better than when he was admitted and little different from a week ago, before he had begun the melphalan.

So when Dr. Sandra Fitzgerald, the transplant unit psychiatrist, paid a visit to Father Greer on Wednesday afternoon, she found him ruddy-complected and alert, his hair neatly combed, seated in a chair by the window and reading his breviary. Their conversation wandered from the Celtics to the weather to a fleeting reference to the extreme nausea he had experienced that morning. As usual, Father Greer treated issues without and within—the problems of the great basketball player Larry Bird's heels as well as the inquietude of his own gastrointestinal tract—with similar equanimity and detachment. And humor. Dr. Fitzgerald was pleased to find him feeling so well, given the assaults his body had already endured, but his bonhomie was even more disconcerting to her than it had been when she had first talked to him months before while interpreting the results of his psychological tests.

Dr. Fitzgerald was, in essence, *the* social service segment of New

England Medical Center's transplant unit. The program was so new, and psychiatric services typically are not given the highest priority when such a group, which deals in physical life and death, is begun within a hospital. Other Boston hospitals, which had been doing transplants for years, had by now taken a more comprehensive approach, utilizing an assortment of social workers, psychiatrists, and psychologists in assisting patients before, during, and following their hospitalizations. Dr. Fitzgerald had been the staff psychiatrist for Dr. Miller's unit for over a year and had worked with more than a dozen transplant patients.

This patient, the first priest she had encountered in her practice, presented her with an unlikely problem: strength. A troublesome, vexing strength.

"I love to see independent men, but he's so *damn* independent," she said as we talked in the hallway outside Father Greer's room. It is not anger, but frustration in her voice. Dr. Fitzgerald is a large, square-shouldered Irish woman with close-cropped hair, no makeup, and a rather stolid expression on her face. Although she seldom smiled, her slow, deliberate manner of speaking somehow conveyed both professional and personal concern.

"The transference almost always takes place," she said. "In other words, the transplant patient projects onto the therapist the expectations and fears of this procedure, likes and dislikes, the deepest feelings that cannot always be revealed to the physicians in charge of his or her case. I am outside that sphere so am usually considered safe to talk to. And because of it, I know how to reach the patient during the worst days in the hospital. It is not too overstated or overdramatic to say the valley of the shadow of death awaits Father Greer and I am no closer to him than I was the first time we met. He is always friendly, courteous, but I sense he senses I am not a person he is going to need.

"The days ahead are going to be horrible. There will be terrible pain; his mouth will be sore beyond anything he is anticipating. He'll be going from both ends. The drugs may well cause psychotic episodes. People sometimes get up and want to walk out of the hospital. I just hope he will eventually trust in me."

That afternoon, Father Greer is taken to the basement of the Proger Building and wheeled into a small room whose three-foot-thick walls are constructed of lead brick. He is helped into the plywood box and forced into a fetal position; his arms are taped to his sides, his legs taped together. Sponges and bags filled with rice, which, because of their density, block the rays, are put in strategic locations at the thinner parts of his body. A Plexiglas sheet is placed over one of the box's open sides and small sheets of lead are carefully positioned to further reduce the amount of radiation that will strike the thinnest parts of his body, such as his head and his lower legs. It is a straightforward procedure: the body is no more than a mass of matter that will absorb a given amount of radiation in a known period of time; it must be irradiated evenly, but thoroughly, half on the right side, half on the left.

Dr. David Wazer, the head of oncological radiation, and his technicians leave the darkened room. Father Greer is alone. Some thirty inches from the box that contains him, a Clinac 2500 linear accelerator, which looks like half of a huge telephone receiver, is silently poised. The only light in the room is emitted from the gantry head of the machine, the square beam delineating the radiation field.

A soft but high-pitched buzzing sound begins. Then there is a duller, muffled roar as the water-cooling system kicks in.

For ten minutes, high-energy photon rays generated by the machine painlessly penetrate Father Greer's body, altering the nuclei of dividing cells, both where the Cytoxan has reached and where it cannot—such areas as the brain and the fluid around it. The cells are not killed outright but mutate and are unable to replicate. The dose of radiation is not strong enough to kill muscle or tissue but is lethal for blood cells and carefully controlled to induce hematological—but not total—death.

Many patients, realizing the gravity of what is happening to their bodies and anticipating the agony that will follow, call out over the intercom to be told how much time they have left. Radiology staff members in the control room watch the patient on a closed-circuit television monitor. Father Greer is silent throughout these first ten minutes and then, after being turned by the technicians, for the ten minutes he is exposed on his left side. He is returned to his room about an hour and a half after leaving it, having received the first two of six doses of 200 rads of radiation.

By the end of the third day and sixth session, Father Greer has been exposed to 1,200 rads. In the Chernobyl nuclear disaster, workers and firemen who were hit with the same amount of radiation were dead within ten days.

As he is being helped out of the plywood box for the last time, Father Greer looks up at the section's coordinator, Cathy Skully.

"Am I well done yet?"

Cards and letters began to arrive, eight, twelve, even twenty a day. And Father Greer read them. Parishioners, fellow priests, old friends sent along good words and prayers, humorous cards with cartoon figures, serious cards with lushly painted bouquets. The phone in his room rang often, everyone from Father Greer's brother, Jim, and sister, Geraldine, to Dom his barber to Cardinal Law, who asked if he might visit, a request Father Greer politely refused, saying he was not feeling well enough. As his bouts of vomiting— and the phone calls—became more frequent, he had the phone disconnected.

On Saturday, the day after he had had his final radiation treatment, I found him lying on top of his neatly made bed, dressed in pajamas and a navy blue robe. He was sleeping peacefully. His color was ruddy and healthy, his breathing steady and slow; he looked like a normally healthy man taking a nap. He had been in the hospital a week. On his bedside table was his breviary, the red ribbon marker at Friday morning's prayer. The text, from Paul's letter to the Galatians, read:

> I have been crucified with Christ, and the life I live now is not my own; Christ is living in me. I still live my human life, but it is a life of faith in the Son of God, who loved me and gave Himself for me.

Father Greer awoke after a half hour, sat up slowly, and shook his head groggily. He smiled weakly, somewhat like a person who had just bumped his head on a familiar beam going into the cellar. He said he was doing his best to fight the nausea, so that he could continue taking solid food and would not have to be totally dependent on intravenous feeding. He laughed as he described being "a mummy" swathed in sterile sheets, with only his eyes showing, on his trips to the radiation room and recounted how hallways and elevators cleared at his approach. "They should have had a bell around my neck," he said. " 'Leper, leper!' they could have called out." Of course, he knew it was just the opposite: the rest of the world held the threat of contamination, not he. Hour by hour his immune system was being destroyed; the ordinary ambient bacteria normal bodies fight off every day were now potentially lethal.

His complaints dispensed within a few terse sentences, he asked about me, my family, the traffic, and "What brings you in to Boston today" as if he were just one casual stop on my list. I asked what had been going through his mind and he was immediately forthcoming.

"I'm fortunate, that's what I've been thinking, happy and lucky to be in here. Everything is going well so far; they tell me I'm tolerating the treatment very well. I'm tired all the time; I can't concentrate well enough to say Mass or to read much anymore, no interest in TV. I'm sick to my stomach and I've got to get up in a few minutes to change my pajamas because this diarrhea has a mind of its own. But I'm lucky to have a chance at a cure. I find myself praying for the sick people in the hospital, people in real pain and people who may not have the faith to get through.

"My faith is in the Lord—yes, in the doctors—but my primary faith is in God. I'm not holding on to this precious treasure called life. I said it to myself before I went into that box for my radiation, when I couldn't think of anything else: 'The Lord is my shepherd, I shall not fear.' I feel very close to God. I can't really pray, but I know that He is in here with me. I know that.

"They're going to let me rest over the weekend, then on Monday I get the transplant. They have to be careful, because that can stop your heart. But I feel ready." His eyelids began to droop and his bottom jaw seemed out of cadence with the upper. "Ready to be reborn."

I left Father Greer in his room, where the music of WJIB was playing on a radio brought down by the blood bank technicians. The walls of the room were bare except for a calendar Sue Tegan had provided and a chart for keeping track of his exercise bicycle miles (Dr. Miller had promised that if he rode 150 miles during his stay, he would be given a free round-trip airplane ticket to anywhere in the world). There was also a small, roughly shaped apple cut from red construction paper by my four-year-old son, Noah. "An apple a day keeps the doctor away," he had said, telling me to pass it on and to insist that the priest post his talisman. Many transplant patients cover their walls with familiar pictures and then the cards and letters they receive, but Father Greer, after looking at his cards, threw them away. He had brought nothing for the walls.

Father Greer believed, echoing the words of St. Paul, that Christ was living within him. At the same time, according to the stack of sixteen-by-twenty-two-inch sheets—his daily flow charts—on a stand outside his door, normal life was abandoning him. His white blood cell count, which had started at 3,500, was now at 800 and would, in a day or two, be zero. His hematocrit—the measure of red blood cells, which live longer than the whites or platelets and which is usually between 35 and 45—was now 32. The short-lived platelets, which allow the blood to clot in a cut or wound, once at a level of 90,000, were now entirely gone.

Father Joseph Greer was fast approaching a certain kind of death. In forty-eight hours, about the same amount of time his Saviour lay in a grave, he was scheduled to begin a certain kind of resurrection, and perhaps a miracle at man's hand.

Shortly after nine o'clock on Monday morning, October 17th, Drs. Miller and Shulman and Sue Tegan enter Father Greer's room. They have scrubbed and wear surgical gowns, rubber gloves, and face masks, as does everyone who enters room 664 now. Dr. Miller usually engages in some small talk before his daily examination of Father Greer; this morning he does not. His face is set, expressionless, his eyes fixed on an immovable point a few feet before him. Rebecca Shulman, who carries herself with an air of authority in the clinic, is clearly the learning assistant in this procedure. She stands off to the side, as if Dr. Miller needs a great amount of room for what he is about to do.

Cradled in Dr. Miller's hand are two oversized syringes, each with a capacity of sixty cubic centimeters. One is full, the other half full of a pale, pinkish liquid. With Father Greer in a partially upright position, leaning back on his pillows, Dr. Miller inserts the needle of the first syringe into a lumen.

While senior members of the transplant team were not known to talk about it, the younger doctors had speculated among themselves what that moment must be like. Dr. Chris Hillyer, whose office in the blood bank was just across the corridor from the room where stem cells and marrow for transplants are stored, wondered, "Is it a neoreligious experience? Think about it: the creation of life. I could see it almost being orgasmic." Rebecca Shulman, reducing the procedure to its theoretical—and to her, most beautiful—minimum, could only think of a single, pleuripotential stem cell floating out of the syringe and into the bloodstream. "It's Adam and Eve all over again; the beginning of life. One cell, just one cell, could do it."

Dr. Miller empties the first syringe in about three minutes. He asks Father Greer how he is feeling and the priest nods; he is fine. As Dr. Miller begins to inject the contents of the second syringe, Father Greer's breathing becomes irregular. His mouth gapes open; he gasps for air. From his mouth comes an overwhelming odor of garlic, which quickly permeates the room. Sue Tegan holds a basin as Father Greer straightens up, dangles his legs over the side of the bed, and vomits. Once they are sure that Father Greer is having no complications other than the nausea, the two doctors leave. Tegan remains.

The peripheral stem cells Father Greer had donated during his long hours in the blood bank that summer had been diluted in saline and DMSO, a preservative, at room temperature the consistency of warm maple syrup. DMSO acts as a sort of shock absorber, filling the delicate crystalline structure of the cells so that the freezing and thawing do not shatter them and render them useless for further reproduction. While DMSO is odorless, as the patient metabolizes it a strong garlic smell is produced in the lungs and is issued forth with each exhalation. Father Greer's reaction to the injection of the stem cells is not uncommon, although intrinsically the solution is not an irritant. It is the smell itself that nauseates the patient.

That afternoon Dr. Hillyer injects the contents of two more bags of stem cells. Father Greer seems to tolerate them better and the transplant team members, pleased with the absence of any major complications or undue discomfort, leave the hospital late in the afternoon. By now they have no reason to believe anything other than that the stem cells are circulating in his blood, some already returning through the porous housing of the bones to resume their natural cycle. There, in the intricate honeycomb that makes up the bone, where marrow once resided with both good cells and the myeloma cells in it, was nothing more than inert, fatty tissue and vacant holes, spaces where life-giving, healthy cells could once again grow.

That evening, Dr. Miller is called by the night nurse on Proger 6 North. Father Greer's blood pressure has unexpectedly soared to 240/120 and the most recent blood lab report shows his creatinine level rising, indicating that his kidneys are beginning to plug up. Dr. Herb Levine, the head of cardiology, is called at home, and a heart monitor is wheeled into room 664 just after midnight. Dr. Miller comes in earlier than usual the next morning and orders the blood bank to thaw the fifth and sixth bags of stem cells, but emphasizes that nothing should be done with the seventh and eighth until they hear from him. That morning Father Greer receives his third round of stem cells.

Immediately thereafter, the key members of the transplant team—Drs. Desforges, Miller, Shulman, and Hillyer—meet to confront a problem they had not anticipated: with each transfusion of stem cells, Father Greer's kidneys are showing increasing levels of creatinine—twice normal—meaning his kidneys are functioning at half their usual rate and are not ridding his body of toxic waste products. Basically, his kidneys are being impeded to a point where further assaults by the body's reaction to the infused solution could shut them down entirely. His bilirubin count is also up; his liver is in distress, and its ability to carry out its task as the body's chemical factory, regulating the sugar level, metabolizing hormones, and detoxifying poisons, is jeopardized.

At the meeting the doctors clash, their combined decades of medical knowledge and experience producing two differing opinions.

The expert clinician Miller says that whatever it is that is causing the problem—he points to the DMSO—should not be risked again with a fourth transfusion. He does not want to chance kidney failure, thus condemning Father Greer to dialysis and a kidney transplant later in addition to the massive assault on his body he is already enduring. Shulman, the most recent medical school graduate but an expert in body chemistry, maintains that nothing in the literature proves DMSO to have this effect. She votes for the fourth transfusion. Earlier studies have shown that marrow transplants given in small doses over an extended period of time are not effective, so if the seventh and eighth bags are not given now, they will probably never be used. Hillyer goes to the phone to call the one person who has more experience with autologous stem cell transplants for multiple myeloma patients than anyone else in the country, Dr. Nancy Kessinger of the University of Nebraska. Dr. Kessinger had just published the first follow-up report on such transplants, based on data from seven patients. It was a small number of scientific standards, but it was all the information at hand.

Hillyer comes back to the group with Dr. Kessinger's opinion. Out of her group of seven, one patient had died of kidney failure after transplant. Whether it was the DMSO or something else that had caused it, she personally would not risk the fourth injection with a patient already experiencing kidney distress. Rebecca Shulman is furious. Dr. Miller again listens to her rationale, finally telling her, raising his voice, "It's something in the bag, something— I don't know what—but it's in the damn bag!" he says, referring to the combined solution of peripheral blood and preservative. "If I was sure what it was, I'd tell you! I'm not." He confers once more with Dr. Desforges and, as the head of the transplant unit, makes the decision.

There will be no fourth transfusion.

Everyone knows this is a technical violation of the protocol the transplant team had written, a breach of their carefully worded criteria that determined who would be accepted and precisely how they would be treated. They had written the protocol with the best information they had at hand, but now, Dr. Miller concludes, it has to be amended for this patient.

Father Greer has received 270 cubic centimeters of stem cells— about a cupful. If the freezing and thawing have not killed more than the usual 30 percent, some 10 million stem cells are within him, with the possibility that they are ordained to, and could, bring him back to life.

6

"Suffer on behalf of others." I whispered this comforting thought to myself all night, but my angel did not return.

It was Sue Tegan who voiced what Father Greer's doctors and the other nursing staff on Proger 6 North had seen so clearly yet had been reluctant to articulate during the first week posttransplant. She stripped off her surgical mask outside room 664, rested her head for an instant on the doorjamb, then looked over at Danny Mc-Clellan, another nurse, who was about to enter 665, the other isolation room. Her voice was laced with the kind of pity staff on high-risk floors like Proger 6 North seldom allow themselves.

"Shouldn't somebody be in there with him?" she pleaded.

Since his admittance more than two weeks before, Father Greer had had no visitors other than hospital personnel. When Father Canniff had called to check on his friend's status, Tegan had told him—though not in graphic detail—of the difficulties Father Greer had begun to experience and had suggested that someone visit him, although the priest from Natick had forbidden this. "He's a private guy," Father Canniff had replied. "When he's ready to see us, he'll let us know."

The answer had not sat well with Tegan. It is not uncommon for a primary nurse to grow close to her patient, to alert family members to needs, and to anticipate mood swings at various stages of the transplant procedure. But for Sue Tegan Father Greer was more than just another man struggling for his life. He was a priest—

Tegan was, as noted, a devout Catholic—and one whom she had immediately liked for his easy good humor and the way he always asked about her as she saw to his needs.

And now, during the worst days a transplant patient endures, he seemed so pitiably alone.

Sue Tegan had an old-fashioned, deep-seated respect for priests stemming from her adolescent years. A young priest in her parish had been especially important to her and had helped her over those teenage years when, among other matters, the survival or demise of religious convictions depends so much on adult role models. She had been nervous when she had learned she would be Father Greer's primary nurse. When she had first touched him to help him dress or to wash him, she was far more tentative than her ten years of experience might have suggested.

Father Greer had sensed this and quickly put her at ease with his ready chatter, his way of saying "Thank you, sweetheart," that conveyed nothing offhanded or familiar but was simply the genuine appreciation of a man who had served so many himself.

But in the last week she had seen that insouciant priest, with a marvelous sense of detachment about himself and his illness, turn bitter and angry. She had witnessed a man of seemingly unshakable faith rage at his doctors, a man of reason become unhinged. She had, with a shaking hand, recorded on his chart Father Greer's words—the first she could understand after days of babbling: "Why did this happen to me? What did I do?"

Sue Tegan, who had both nursed people back to life and prepared them for death, was terrified.

He was not a patient who confided in her deeply, as many do, so all she could judge by were the externals—and her imagination. The externals were grim enough. His creatinine level was slowly dropping, and although the guarded opinion on the floor was that he had passed through that danger, his bilirubin count was still high, indicating liver trouble. With a dysfunctional immune system, there was a constant risk of developing hepatitis. And then there were what are considered the "normal" side effects of a transplant, of a magnitude only a patient can ever know.

In his mouth and down through the long and winding tube that is the human gastrointestinal tract, pieces of dead tissue had peeled off, leaving behind raw sores. His mouth was bubbly with a herpes infection, his throat swollen. Saliva, properly generated but now with no place to go, streamed out of the corners of his mouth. His joints ached. His stomach churned and lapsed into painful spasms. And his mind, that most precious and, according to Catholic teaching from Augustine to Aquinas, ultimately controllable organ, which his rigorous schooling and priestly life had trained to hold sway over whatever the problem or temptation, had gone awry.

Father Greer could not read, could not concentrate long enough to recite the 23rd Psalm, which he had last said, over and over when he could think of nothing else, as he sat crammed inside the tiny plywood box, his body bombarded with photons.

"The Lord is my shepherd. . . . The Lord is. . . . The Lord . . ." And then blankness, a horrifying blankness. The needle of his consciousness would not lift from the groove in which he was stuck. A man who had never suffered from headaches and who thought the pain he had experienced in Scotland was unbearable now felt the jaws of a vice tightening at his temples. The physical pain throughout his body was far more acute than he had anticipated, many times more intense than he had ever felt before, but the true agony—for a man who had always prided himself on his rationality—was the loss of his reason. The morphine and Ativan had induced a dreamlike state, the antihistamines and antibiotics, antiinflammatories and steroids, the antiviral agents, all swirling about in a pharmacological witch's brew, had assaulted his central nervous system. The synapses of the electrical impulses that normally convey thought patterns and sensations were short-circuiting.

He had read articles about bone marrow transplants and talked to others who had undergone the treatment, but now, in his semilucid moments, he knew that the reports from this battlefront had been so much revisionist fiction.

Further, Father Greer was hallucinating: There was a recurring and gruesome accident. Sometimes he was the victim, sometimes not—equally a punishment to have to watch and not be able to help. The twisted wreckage, the body bloody and limp. Over and over, the impact, the sound, the carnage. The hallucination dragged on. He waited for help to come. No one did.

And then there were the dogs. The cats.

The accident victim turned into a huge, vicious dog. Father Greer could smell it, feel its hot breath, see the snarling jaws, the huge teeth. The dog was suddenly *there* in the room, prowling about, ominous, bigger, more vicious, still more huge—but always silent, and the silence of the beast added to its savagery. Father Greer felt the floor shudder with the weight of this enormous creature. He saw the paw prints on his sheets.

A fastidious man who disliked clutter in his rectory kitchen or on the altar, Father Greer had always had an enormous distaste for dogs. He had found even more reason to hate them while working as a postman during his college years. Now dogs with muscular shoulders, huge heads, and glaring eyes were defying him to so much as move. And cats; he would do anything to avoid touching them. Now they were coming to haunt and taunt him. Cats of monstrous size stalked in front of his bed, arrogant in their slow, deliberate pace.

Each time they came to haunt him, he sat up in bed with a start, drenched with perspiration, his sore-encrusted mouth screaming for water.

Coming out of the hallucination, his momentarily semilucid mind scrambled to grasp its moorings. It was the Agony in the Garden, the night before the Crucifixion, and like the disciples he could not stay awake long enough to pray or be present for the man who was going to be sacrificed. Prayer? He needed desperately to pray, his beclouded mind commanded him to, but he could not. His body was crying out so loud no voice could be raised above it. God was far away.

It was not a matter of transcendence as he had foretold; he could think only of preservation.

In his delirium, Father Greer knew he needed his Saviour more than anything, that He was the only safeguard against these demons and against the unforgivable sin: despair. The Holy Eucharist, his Saviour, the One who had stood against the forces of the netherworld and triumphed. There was no thought of saying Mass—his Mass kit, the bottle of wine, unopened since his arrival, mocked him from the closet. But the Eucharist, at least that.

His throat was swollen shut from the herpes. Nothing would pass.

"Though I walk through the valley . . . the valley . . . the valley . . ."

It was not all hallucination. Indeed, he had been in an accident. He had experienced a collision; his body was in shock. He had lost his life-sustaining blood, just as that battered victim in his mind had done. But his collision was, for the time being, at the forefront of science, as carefully controlled a procedure as medical knowledge could provide, yet a gross example of overkill, a late-twentieth-century equivalent of boring holes in the head to relieve pain, of bleeding a patient to cleanse the blood.

At times he grabbed at his neck because of the searing pain. He would vomit three, four, as many as seven or eight times a shift, gagging, almost suffocating as he forced air down his swollen windpipe. He had constant diarrhea. His temperature soared to over 104. When he rolled over—painfully—clumps of his fine hair were left behind in the indentation of the pillow.

Sue Tegan held a straw in a cup of cool water, but he could not swallow a sip. Father Greer gazed at her forlornly. "Just to think," he rasped, "I took it all for granted. I can't even do this."

On his windowsill were two huge piles of newly arrived cards and letters. He had neither the strength to open nor the will to read them.

Dr. Miller visited each morning and assured Father Greer that this was all normal—the temperature because he had no white blood cells to fight infection, the sores, nausea, and diarrhea because the soft lining within his body had been scoured. Everything was going exactly as it should. And had to.

Even when he was finally able to speak, Father Greer often said nothing in return.

After one visit, Dr. Miller lingered outside Father Greer's room, as if somehow his presence outside would bring the comfort he could not impart in person. "I hate it every time," he said. The priest had spoken this time, to lash out at the physician that it was "immoral" to promise that trip to any transplant patient who could log 150 miles on the exercise bicycle. "You keep on saying to yourself that you cannot cross over the line between being the doctor and a concerned human being—a friend—but I would be a fool to stand here and say I can keep a distance during these days," he said. "In the seven to ten days after transplant you are uniquely close to your patient. It is a risky, extraordinarily painful procedure; he feels like he's being choked. Except for pain medication and antibiotics for the infection, we have little control. All we can do is wait for the stem cells to engraft and hope that he doesn't get an infection so severe we can't treat it.

"Regardless of the potential benefits, there is a fact I cannot escape, and I don't get any better at this. I did that to that man in there," he said, pointing through room 664's window to the form lying on the bed, his back to the door. "I have taken him to a point of no return. Can I bring him out the other side?

"The man could die. He might never walk out of that room." He turned abruptly and walked rapidly away, tearing off his rubber gloves and surgical gown.

Sue Tegan felt ever more helpless as the days passed and still the priest had no visitors. She considered calling Father Canniff or Father Greer's sister or brother, but when she asked the priest if she might do so, he would not allow it. "Listen, I want to get a little better before I see anyone," he snapped, angry at her for asking. "Understand?"

The large flow charts outside his room recorded how much liquid was entering his body intravenously, how much waste was being expelled, his temperature, his pulse, blood pressure, the levels of calcium, albumin, neutrophils—some twenty-two indicators of body chemistry, including his white blood cell count, which was still zero. Tegan, the other nurses, and the doctors who visited him—Desforges, Shulman, and Miller—all entered more personal observations on his chart. But there was little to say that was not repetitive.

What the chart did not say plainly was the major fact: there was a sick, sullen, angry man in room 664.

One doctor was absent, and during this pivotal week her observations might have cast the most light on what Father Greer was experiencing. Sandy Fitzgerald had contracted pneumonia, and even when she returned to limited service at the medical center, she would not be able to enter his room for some time—for fear of infecting him.

7

If you want to love don't place yourself beyond love's reach.

Jackie Forest* was the patient in 665, the other isolation room, next to Father Greer's. Although he had not seen her (she had been in posttransplant toxic shock when he was admitted) he knew that she was young—twenty, to be exact—engaged—her fiancé was a frequent visitor and could often be seen in the hallway—and had Hodgkin's disease. The nurses and doctors who entered Father Greer's room, while being careful to carry neither the bacteria nor the distress of the outside world, daily brought him news of Proger 6 North, albeit selectively, conveying only the most positive reports of a hospital floor where there is far more tragedy than triumph.

As he lay in bed in an agony that showed no sign of abating, Father Greer knew within the hour when the signal event occurred: Jackie Forest had taken her first steps outside her room. Her white blood cell count had risen above 1,000 and she had, however minimally, regained the ability to withstand infection. Her marrow was engrafting. The step from room to hallway is one every transplant patient knows is as important and crucial as any he or she will ever make. It is the bridge between the protected environment of germ-free isolation and the real world.

But on this momentous occasion Father Greer still did not know what Jackie Forest looked like.

Forest was one of three young women Dr. Miller had treated in the past month, which he had termed "the worst month in my medical career." All three, he said of them affectionately, were "femmes fatales," attractive, vivacious young women whom he and his photons and array of cell killers had leveled. Forest, who just a month before had had a full head of radiant auburn hair, a strong, upright way of walking, was now a wraithlike creature with bulging eyes, no hair, a shuffling, unsure walk—a woman who could have passed for sixty if seen from a distance, pushing her IV pole on wheels through the corridor of Proger 6 North.

That same day, in the "WBC" column on the chart outside Father Greer's door, where a series of zeros had been entered for the past week, there was a change. Sue Tegan, taking the number from the blood lab report, recorded 100. She burst into the room—after a quick scrub and donning her protective clothing—to tell Father Greer but quickly injected a note of caution. Sometimes, she told him bluntly, the lab can "screw up" and give an indication of a white blood cell count—100 is the lowest amount the lab can measure—when there actually is none. And if the count is real, it can just as easily drop the next day. But she wanted to give her patient some reason to smile again; it had been so long. "You're on your way!" she said, her gloved hand on his shoulder.

Father Greer received the news without the slightest show of emotion. His temperature, which had been successfully controlled by three different antibiotics in the first few days after his transplant, had again spiked at 102. There had been so little to measure in his recovery during the last week, but at least he had felt he had beaten the temperature. And now, as his mind began to clear and the beasts of his hallucinations to retreat, Father Greer saw his elevated temperature as a serious setback. He lay in his bed hour after hour, a cool paper cloth on his forehead, his jaw grimly set. He did not want to watch television or have the radio on. He was not reading anything. His breviary and a growing mound of cards—the stacks had collapsed into each other—sat on the windowsill. The only envelope he had opened was his absentee ballot, which he had filled out with Tegan's help.

He was sleeping poorly. The lack of total rest—a few hours, or were they only minutes, he couldn't tell—of rest kept him in exhausted bondage. He had developed a body rash, angry clusters of tiny red bumps on his torso, hands, and arms that were constantly

itching. His throat and mouth were so much raw flesh that even
the gentle breeze of ordinary inhalation hurt. He had been taken
off morphine, and unlike many transplant patients who beg to return
to the semistupor it produces, the priest had wanted no more. Sue
Tegan had encouraged him to ask for the drug if the pain was
unbearable; she knew there was no reason for transplant patients to
suffer unduly or to remember what they have endured. The priest
said no.

To Sue Tegan he was a stoic, a martyr, a consecrated priest in
a hospital dickey stained with drool and the uncontrollable moisture
of his bowels. But on the afternoon of his first white blood cell
count he became something else. With a simple confession he
became a man, hurting, who needed her.

"We take so many things for granted," he said to her almost
involuntarily, as if he could keep the words in no longer, the tone
of his voice depleted of any feeling. "I took so many things for
granted." And Tegan could see that although he had allowed no
member of his family, no friend, no fellow priest to comfort him,
he was, for the first time, reaching out for emotional support.

It continued. The gestures were small but sure.

"I would be ready to leave the room after helping him with his
bath, or sitting with him on the edge of the bed, and he would ask
me to move the box of tissues closer," she said a few days later,
reflecting on the change. "Or to fix one of the blinds on the window.
Or to fluff up his pillow. Or to fold down the blankets. It was
obvious he just wanted to keep me in the room, but he never said,
'Sue, just stay here for a while.' But that's what he wanted; I could
see it. Each time I left, I assured him I'd be back in fifteen minutes
or a half hour. And I stuck to it. When you're in that isolation
room, every minute drags by. He was lonely.

" 'I feel so sick; when is this going to get better?' he would say
to me, knowing there was no quick answer but that I would listen
to him every time he said it. Doctors are in and out of the room
in minutes; a nurse can afford to take time. I could see by the look
on his face the pain he was in, but then he'd ask me to help him
sit up or to take a few steps in the room. Some patients just lie back;
he is a fighter. Some are so self-involved with their pain; he is always
aware of the person serving him.

"He's the kind of patient who wants to suffer alone, I think, because he wants to make sure it won't hurt others to see him like he is. He has an idea of who he is and what he is and he isn't that person now and he doesn't want people seeing him this way. His role is his life, I guess, and it's hard for him to slip out of it. Everyone depended on him, and now he is dependent on us. But if he only knew how wonderful it is to be needed by someone like him, he might let others in. From the calls I get and the cards that come in, he has so many people who love him. I guess in me he sees someone who isn't family and isn't a doctor, someone neutral in a way and whose job it is to care for him. This is my *job*. That makes sense; he can give in to that."

In these dark days another member of the hospital staff also reached him: not the motherly Dr. Desforges or the expert clinician Dr. Miller, who was ultimately directing his case, not Carol or Lisa or Allen who visited him from the blood bank, but the newest and least experienced person on the transplant team.

She was as reserved and private a person as he, and the priest reminded her so much of her own taciturn father. Out of these similarities Rebecca Shulman began to forge a bond with Father Greer that was unspoken but deeply felt. It was Dr. Shulman who could make the priest smile even after he had presented a stern face to the senior doctors who had just left the room. Dr. Shulman's own serious, even dour, face seemed transformed by her visits to room 664. She wrote on his flow chart with her head cocked to the side, a look on her face as if she were listening to a favorite Beethoven sonata and not recording her observations of a man teetering between life and death. Rebecca Shulman, whose emotional state was as much of a mystery to the hematology/oncology staff as the elusive pleuripotential stem cell was, actually looked happy after seeing Father Greer.

She was now a few months pregnant, and Father Greer knew before most of her colleagues did.

First it was a single swallow of room-temperature orange juice. Then a fraction of a teaspoon of melting raspberry sherbet. A few ounces of water. Apple juice. And on the twelfth day posttransplant, Father Greer told Sue Tegan to make sure the Catholic chap-

lain, Father Edmund Charest, stopped by room 664 on his daily
rounds. Father Greer had been forced to forgo, for the longest period
in his adult life, a nourishment he had thought about so often and
hungered for during his delirium. Now, finally, his throat was ready.
He could swallow without choking.

Throughout the worst days, it had seemed that if he only could
receive Holy Communion, the confusion and pain would be less,
but even in his disordered state, he had been aware enough not to
risk asking his God to enter his body, only to have to spit Him out.

"The Body of Christ." Father Charest held a sliver of a Host—
no more than a tenth of one—before Father Greer's lips, still swollen
and blistered with the herpes infection. He placed the particle on
Father Greer's inflamed and crusted tongue. Father Greer carefully
coaxed it to the back of his mouth and cautiously swallowed.

The sense of relief was immediate.

All Father Greer could think of was that he had swallowed solid
food.

Father Greer was soon able to sit unaided with his legs over the
side of his bed. He could walk the ten or twelve steps to the shower
without hesitating for rest. After being out of his bed for any period
of time, he returned to it utterly exhausted and found he was unable
to so much as roll over for the next half hour or so, but he was
beginning to move about in his room more or less independently.

On the chest-high stand outside room 664, increasingly larger
amounts of liquids were listed under "Oral" on his flow chart, and
in the "WBC" column a steadily rising figure indicated that the
bone marrow, which had been killed, was indeed now alive and
producing white blood cells: 100, 200, 300, 100, 200, 400, 400.
The rise was slow but generally steady. The resurrection was being
documented.

While his blood counts continued to climb ("Everything's right
within the normal range" his doctors assured him daily, noting, in
fact, that the white count had returned as early as they had ever
seen), another of the lab tests that monitors the body chemistry of
a transplant patient gave cause for serious concern. Father Greer's
bilirubin count, 1.8, indicated that his liver function was still impaired. Either a latent strain of hepatitis had found an opportunity

to flourish in Father Greer's immune-suppressed body, or the powerful drugs had inflamed and blocked the liver's ducts.

There was nothing to do but wait for the lining to heal naturally—no medication could heal it—and a judgment was made not to burden him with this problem by telling him about it. Dr. Desforges, who is normally so straightforward with patients, telling them the exact magnitude of their disease and their prospects, said, "Frankly, at a time like this I don't believe in *that* kind of truth."

Father Greer finally allowed his brother, Jim, who is two years younger, and his sister, Geraldine, who is ten years younger, to visit. Yet when Cardinal Law called again and wanted to come by, Father Greer asked him to "give me a little more time to get my socks on." He was too weak to climb up on the exercise bike, but he did begin to look at the mountain of mail that had accumulated. He read the names, the shortest notes, and the first paragraph or so of the longer ones before dropping them into the brown paper bag at his bedside. He watched most of the first quarter of the Notre Dame–Boston College game before falling asleep. Last year he had been in South Bend for this Catholic classic.

Later that week, on Saturday, November 5, the eighteenth day posttransplant, Dr. Kenneth Miller stood before the chart outside Father Greer's room. In front of him was a success story of modern medicine: a man who had been hematologically dead a little over two weeks before had a rising white blood cell count—now 1.6, or 1600—normal temperature, an acceptable bilirubin count of .6, and an "Oral" column jammed with Popsicles, ginger ale, cola, and juices—the information sometimes annotated with smiling faces the nurses had drawn in. There had been no major infections, no uncontrolled bleeding. Father Greer had left the room for his first short walk in the corridor the day before. Visitors no longer had to dress in surgical gowns and rubber gloves—just a mask—to enter his room. In many respects he was ready to be released from the hospital. In all probability he would leave in a few days, about three weeks after being reinfused with his stem cells. It had been a remarkably quick recovery.

"It didn't work," Dr. Miller said, shaking his head as he made an entry.

He turned. His normally sharp features were muted, his eyes, usually in constant motion surveying what is going on about him—the eyes of a basketball player—were still, downcast. "I thought he would go inside for strength, but he didn't. Physically, he is doing wonderfully. Beyond our expectations. Mentally, he is in a crushing depression. Frankly, it's shocking in its intensity. No matter what I say, he's not listening. I mentioned to him that his seminary training must have prepared him to be alone like this. He said, 'I flunked that part.' His faith . . ." the doctor hesitated, a precise man now dealing with an imponderable, ". . . his faith just didn't click in for him.

"He expects to feel better immediately, and we know that he will not. He's able to take solid foods, and in celebration of that last night he ordered chicken divan. He vomited an hour later. He's in there trying to drive himself to feel better and do more and get out of here quicker than anybody, but he can't do it, can't control the situation with an act of the will as he is used to doing. He is very, very angry.

"Most transplant patients go to their family for support. I thought his church was his family and he would depend on them. But he is alone, choosing to be alone, and there is a terrible sadness about him. The risky part of the transplant is largely over; the bone marrow does its work without any prodding. The mind doesn't. There are a lot of rough days yet ahead for him. I don't want him leaving the hospital in that state of mind to go to some rectory where there is really no one to care for him. No one to care for that *part* of him.

"It's strange: most patients are shocked by the specifics of the transplant procedure before they go in; they really don't hear you. You can tell by the vacant look in their eye that you are tuned out. They need that denial just to get them into the room. Father Greer listened and understood. Why not now?

"Somehow he feels he failed, that he wasn't strong enough during the time when he was very, very sick. That he lost it. Hell, everybody loses it! We almost kill a person, what are they supposed to do but lose it? He lost control, and it's eating him up. Somehow he wasn't supposed to show anything. Somehow we weren't supposed to know how sick he was. Every time I ask him what is or was the biggest problem—and when he's willing to answer me—it's always about losing control."

Later that morning, Father Greer allowed me into his room for a short visit. It was the first time since transplant day.

I had been sitting quietly in a corner of the room on that crucial day. Suddenly, just as he was being injected with the solution containing the stem cells, he shouted, "No more questions!" Of course, I had not been asking him anything. I left immediately.

He knew I had been visiting the hospital regularly, but since that day I had caught only glimpses of him through the window in his door.

When I entered the room, he was seated on his bed, his legs over the side. A normally erect man, he was again slouched over, as if the weight of his shoulders were more than he could tolerate. I pulled a chair around in front of him so he would not have to turn, but he would not so much as look at me, preferring to stare out the window. By now, he had lost most of his hair. All that remained was a sparse stand of whitish-grey hair, thin and disconcertingly long. His eyes, which, as I had learned over the months, customarily assumed that mournful hound's look when he was confronted with the foibles of ordinary mortals, were filmy and bloodshot. And unmistakably sad. He had aged years in the days he had spent in room 664.

I thought I knew him reasonably well and that we had developed a trust through our many months together. I had always felt comfortable with him, even when he was in a quiet mood and saying little. But this was different. Not knowing what to say, I nervously recited the physical results of his lab tests as an affirmation of his recovery, but I could tell all I was doing was annoying him. I forecasted that if his recovery proceeded at the same pace as during these two weeks, he would be back at St. Patrick's—as he had always planned—by Easter.

He finally looked at me, his face tightening and his Adam's apple bobbing as he swallowed to control his nausea. "I couldn't even eat a piece of toast this morning; that's how great I'm doing."

I reiterated how well the doctors had said he was progressing and that his appetite would soon come back. Suddenly he cut me off. "Your mind does funny things," he blurted out. "I'm not the same guy I was a month ago. I know who came in this joint. But who's leaving? St. Patrick's? I don't know."

I tried to dispel that, but he again stopped me, snapping, "I've got enough doctors around here. I don't need another one."

I knew he wanted me to leave. And then, strangely, he began to talk. "You're a neuter in here. I was in a vacuum, like being drunk for two weeks. Intellect and will—what distinguishes us from animals—were taken away from me. And like St. Peter in the garden, I fell on my face. I'd said, 'God, if it is Your will that I be cured, I'll thank You. If this my cross, I'll take it.'

"So many words. So many hollow, meaningless words."

Sandra Fitzgerald, who by now had recovered from her pneumonia but still had a cold and couldn't enter Father Greer's room, explained as best she could a patient she admitted she did not know well: "He is at a very unfortunate juncture in the life of a transplant patient. His mind is no longer confused by drugs; he is well enough to think. And to remember how horrible it was and realize he may have bought the ranch. He made a decision and now can't turn back, and he's wondering if it was worth it. Of course, it's a question no one can answer—not even him right now. The room is closing in on him. He's a driven man, but he can't concentrate long enough to get anything but the simplest task done. He's angry he's not out yet, and he's equally afraid of leaving because of the increased risk of infection outside the hospital."

After my visit with Father Greer I stopped at St. Patrick's rectory to tell the staff about their pastor. Janet Hamilton, the church secretary, said he had called her a few days before and asked about a few items of church business but then had quickly wanted to end the conversation. She had asked him who would be looking after him when he went to St. Mary's parish in Charlestown. It was a concern not only of Hamilton, but of many of the women who knew Father Greer well, the current and former parishioners closest to him.

"I'll have two priests there," Father Greer had answered her.

"Yes?" was Hamilton's reply, implying she was less than impressed.

Father Rossi, who well knew the dark side of Father Greer from the early days of the multiple myeloma diagnosis, promised to write a long and positive letter. Father Moritz, who by now had moved into Father Greer's room, seemed not to have heard the psychological report but concentrated on the positive medical aspects.

Dolly the housekeeper was beaming, regardless of what she was hearing. She had had a dream the night before. She had been buffing the bannister in the front hall with furniture polish and Father Greer had come through the front door. She hadn't stopped to put down the polish and had run toward him, telling him how good it was to have him back.

He had looked fit and healthy. And he had been hungry, ready for dinner.

8

A terrible night. No sooner had I shut my eyes than desolation came upon me. I can find no other word to describe this indefinable exhaustion, as though my very soul were bleeding to death. I awoke with a start, with a loud cry ringing in my ears. But was it really a cry? Is that the word for it? No, obviously.

"He talks about being changed," said Dr. Jane Desforges. "Yes, Father Greer has been changed. All transplant patients are. At least temporarily. They faced death. In a sense, they *were* clinically dead. But they came back. And after that, a person reevaluates everything. Very few transplant patients go back to doing what they did before. They seem to select what they enjoy doing and no longer do things out of a sense of duty. Years ago Father Greer chose and accepted a role in life. He will have to choose it again, if he is to continue functioning as a parish priest. Only he will be able to decide. Physically, he'll be able. I would see him better in about three months, one hundred days posttransplant.

"We know so much about his physical state, his body chemistry, but Father Greer walks out of the hospital today a man who was given insights during those days in his room that none of us can fathom. I have not endured the fright he did, the sensation induced by all the medication. The vulnerability that one false step, one infection could end his life. I didn't lose my free will. What he discovered about himself and what those insights result in, no one can tell.

"But we learned from him. We learned that we expected too much of Father Greer. We somehow expected him to be different from other patients, to be able to handle this horrible procedure in some superhuman fashion. We expected him to be above the fray. It doesn't work that way. When people are sick, it is so biological, so overwhelmingly biological, that the spiritual aspects, the spiritual recovery, must wait."

Dr. Desforges sat in her office at the New England Medical Center. She had just spent much more time than usual in room 664 as Father Greer prepared to leave. She was struck not only by the confession he had made to her this morning—that he had been weak—but with the intensity with which it had been presented.

In response, Dr. Desforges had gone back to the day Father Greer couldn't get up from the floor in St. Patrick's rectory because of the severe pain in his back. Detail by detail, she had gone over his medical history with him, as well as the history of treatment for multiple myeloma, assuring him that he had not only not been weak, but had been exceedingly brave. She impressed upon him that what had been done was necessary—as best she knew—for him to have any chance at total remission. Without that walk through the valley of the shadow of death, he would have had no chance of survival.

The threat of infection, of contracting pneumonia, of the bone marrow not being able to produce the complex variety of cells Father Greer would need to lead a normal life—these were all worrisome considerations for Dr. Desforges. But foremost in her mind as she returned to her office after rounds was a question medical science could not answer. Who would be there immediately and consistently for Father Greer in the days ahead, when he would be aboard a roller coaster of emotions and symptoms? Dr. Desforges had been accustomed to family members and friends of transplant patients visiting or calling, inquiring about their status while in the hospital, asking how they best could help in the recovery period.

No one had called on Father Greer's behalf.

If Dr. Desforges felt frustrated by her inability to convince Father Greer of his steadfastness—an unusual lament in itself—the patient himself was positively crestfallen. His confinement was supposed to have led to deeper spirituality, to contemplation. His suffering was to have identified him with the agony of his Saviour. But all he had felt was raw pain and numbing confusion, not transcendence. Was it weakness or hubris? Father Greer did not know, but he had no sense of spiritual insight, of any kind of accomplishment, no identification with anyone other than his feeble mortal self.

He was leaving the hospital, free perhaps of the myeloma but, he believed, only a shell of the man who had entered thirty-one days before. He had trouble concentrating on even the most routine task; he could not read more than a few lines before lapsing into some disengaged state of mind. Before his transplant, he had wanted nothing more than to return to his parish, to give whatever years he had left of his life to the duties he had successfully performed in his thirty years as a priest.

He was no longer sure he wanted or would ever be able to return to St. Patrick's.

"This thing up here," Father Greer said, pointing at his head as we talked later in room 664, "has got to clear. I don't know what's been done to me. I don't know what's left." His eyes were red, which they had often been during his stay in the hospital, but also moist, disclosing a vulnerability I had not witnessed before. And for a man whose complexion is normally so ruddy, he looked extraordinarily pale.

As he sat in a chair by the window dressed in trousers and shirt, he looked somehow adrift on a body of water he could not navigate. He mumbled something about being very depressed that morning. He appeared to be ready to cry. He looked away and cleared his throat, and when he turned back to me moments later the old control was back.

"I know that the X rays made me sterile and that I need new glasses and, if I live that long, I'll need a cataract operation in a couple of years. I know the range of possibilities out there. A woman who had a transplant two years ago still has to get transfusions of platelets every ten days. There is a guy who went back to work five weeks after his. Some leave their hospital room on a stretcher with a sheet over their face. My recovery started early, but it didn't exactly take off. I'm not producing any platelets. I have to come in twice a week to get platelets and red blood cells. I'll just have to see.

"Leaving is more important than arriving right now." His face took on a quizzical look, as if he had just uttered a koan, in which the meaning of every word is obvious but the message remains elusive.

Father Greer left the hospital able to keep down such solid foods as farina, dry toast, and applesauce; his white blood cell count was an acceptable 1.6. His level of neutrophils, immature white blood cells that are key infection fighters, was low, but his kidney and liver functions were close to normal. He had been meticulous in the care of his mouth, using soft sponges on sticks instead of a toothbrush, which could have caused bleeding, and scrupulous about cleaning the area around his anus. Both ends of the human pipeline, exposed to air and tissue breakdown, are prime targets for infection when immunity is suppressed. His final checkup that morning had shown Father Greer to be clear of any irritation.

Father Greer was given a partial bill as he signed out: $69,000, not including physicians' fees and numerous other costs. Before the transplant, he had been advised that the procedure would eventually cost about $130,000. He had notified the Archdiocese of Boston of the impending costs and had been assured that his medical insurance coverage was adequate.

Father Greer's destination was a newly refurbished and heartily scrubbed suite of three rooms on the third floor of St. Mary's rectory in Charlestown. The rectory, a warren of small rooms that hearken back to days when the church was staffed by five priests and might have two or three more in residence, was now home to a pastor—his good friend, Father James Canniff—and a part-time assistant, Father Robert Burns, who was studying for his doctorate at Boston University. The rectory was an imposing red brick Boston town house overlooking the grassy knoll of Monument Square and the famous obelisk within it, the Bunker Hill Monument. St. Mary's rectory had a part-time housekeeper and cook, more than sufficient, as Father Greer saw it, to attend to his needs.

Although the three flights of stairs from his rooms to the main-floor dining room exhausted him, Father Greer forced himself to make the trip for most meals. Likewise he forced himself to eat—small portions of overcooked vegetables, dry bread, pudding. He had no appetite, really, and no sense of taste, and he was often nauseated. On the fourth day he ventured out of the rectory alone and managed to walk several hundred feet up the sidewalk and return. By the end of the first week he was able to walk the quarter mile around Monument Square. He had set up an altar in his room but did not yet feel strong enough to say Mass, even with Father Canniff assisting him.

On the tenth day Father Greer was back in the hospital.

A herpes infection had developed in his rectal area, and because his immune system was still suppressed, it had quickly flared out of control. Dr. Desforges admitted the priest for a few days, so that antibiotics stronger than those he routinely took could be administered intravenously. Just after Father Greer was admitted, Dr. Desforges came into room 664—which had been vacant since he left—wondering what frame of mind she would find him in. She was both surprised and pleased to see him greet her with a rather resigned, but nonetheless full-fledged grin. Acting upon her instincts that Father Greer should have something to do in the hospital that would make him, in some small way, less of a patient, she asked if a group of medical students might visit to speak with him about his transplant.

Father Greer agreed and when the seven students came to his room the next morning he told them first of all not to believe anything that had been written from the transplant patient's point of view, that no one undergoing the procedure could accurately remember what went on in the worst days. Then he related in detail exactly what had happened to him. His tale captivated the students.

"I was self-assured," he told them. "Then the tables were turned. When the depression comes on you, you've got to believe in another power. During the worst parts, I kept repeating the Twenty-third Psalm over and over. And what a blessing it was, depending on God. I just hope I carry that dependence with me outside this room."

"It's a new Father Greer," Dr. Desforges said, beaming. "When he smiles, those wonderful wrinkles are back at the corners of his eyes."

The roller coaster was at a peak.

Still another Father Greer descended the stairs at St. Mary's a week later, an antacid lozenge visible on his tongue, a contorted look on his face that to me was shocking because of the pain it showed. He eased into a chair as if every joint in his body were riddled with rheumatism. He did not look at me. He did not want to talk. He had thought of calling to say he didn't want to see me anymore. He wasn't sleeping, and in his sleeplessness he had concluded that our working together was a major part of the problem. "I don't want to think about anything but getting better," he said.

He was not getting better, he went on; in fact, he felt worse than when he had initially been released from the hospital. He was having to go into the hospital twice weekly for massive transfusions of red blood cells and platelets.

As for his future, he held out little hope that he would ever return to St. Patrick's or function as a parish priest.

More than once he mentioned the "one hundred days" during which the bone marrow of the transplant patient should again resume full function. It was his impression that unless this happened by the end of those days he would have to face a reinfusion of his stored marrow, which certainly contained myeloma cells. He appeared fixated on that number: one hundred days.

He was now some forty days posttransplant and held little hope he would make the cutoff date.

"I'm freezing," he said as he slowly rose from his seat in the small, dimly lit parlor on the rectory's second floor. He was wearing a shirt, sweatshirt, and sweater. The knitted cuffs of his pajama bottoms were visible at his trouser cuffs. "I have to get back to bed."

At a time like this, confronted with somebody as sick as Father Greer, it was not difficult for me to believe him and accept some complicity in hindering his recovery. Something I was doing or saying had to be horribly wrong.

I was not the only person questioning the role he or she might be playing in Father Greer's life. When I called Janet Hamilton, the church secretary, to tell her of Father Greer's sudden turn, she said she might have the reason for it.

"Father Greer called the other day, asked how things were going, and I guess I might have complained a bit about what I was doing, having to call the plumber and deal with the cemetery workers and make sure there were enough small Hosts on the altar so the big ones wouldn't have to be broken up. We have four grown men here

in the rectory; what were they doing? This was the kind of stuff
Father Greer always handled himself. 'You better get back,' I told
him. He just laughed and said 'Don't wait for me.'

"I don't know how the conversation switched around, but he
asked how John Craig was doing. John was the brother of a priest
friend and had cancer. He and his wife and Father Greer had dinner
together during the summer and got to be pretty close, both of them
sick as they were. I'd forgotten that Father Greer didn't know about
what happened. So like a fool I just let it out: 'Didn't you know?
He died the day you were admitted. Father Mullaney buried him.'
Of course he didn't know. But what could I say? I felt so rotten.
There was this long pause on the line and Father Greer said he had
to go. I sure didn't help him out that time."

Sandra Fitzgerald had other insights based on her work with other
transplant patients. "Inability to sleep, endless rumination, and the
inability to concentrate—the classic signs of clinical depression.
What brings it on? No one can imagine the horrors of that isolation
room. And now, weeks after, they are in limbo. There is nothing
exciting or momentous, like the actual transplant, to look forward
to; rather, the dailiness of their lives and the slow recovery. They
cannot turn back, and they don't know if they will ever have a
future. They keep on asking: was it worth it? And we have no good
answer.

"In Father Greer, we have a man who has overcome many things
by sheer willpower. He is a man of great strength. An individualist.
But throughout his life he never let anyone into the deepest part of
his soul. Now he may have entered that part, and it may terrify
him. We don't know—and he may not consciously know. He relied
on no one, asked no family member or friend to be with him when
he was in there puking his guts out. He has always relied on himself,
and now he may be wondering who 'himself' is."

A week later, Janet Hamilton looked out the window and was
astonished to see a man in a green paper surgical mask and a funny-
looking peaked fur hat slowly get out of a car on the street near the
kitchen entrance to St. Patrick's. Once inside the kitchen, he took
off his coat and hat. "Don't have much to show," he said, referring
to his head, now almost entirely bald.

He looked so tired, she thought, and old. She noticed he still had thick hair on his forearms. He sat, regaining his breath, and looked around him at the devastation of a kitchen in the early stages of renovation. He offered no comment on it. "Good to be out; needed to walk around a little bit," he said.

He had come, he told her, "for some books," but when he went up to his suite, all he retrieved was the breviary for this, the first quarter of the liturgical year, which began with Advent. He seemed not to be troubled by the fact that Father Moritz, having found the third-floor guest room too small, had moved into his suite. He sat at his desk for a few minutes. Father Moritz had left everything on the desk as it was out of respect for the pastor on leave.

When he came downstairs, Father Greer took out a slip of paper. Janet Hamilton tried to mask her pleasure as he went down the list: Was the lease for the parking lot back from the chancery so it could be signed by the Town of Natick? What about the gutters on the convent? How was the clearing of the boulders in the cemetery going? But he showed no inclination either to offer advice or to reassert any control in the parish. He put on his hat and jacket. He had difficulty getting the zipper started, and Janet helped him.

"So?" she said.

"So what?" he answered.

"So how is it going?"

"The hundred days; ain't going to make that one. Had a little nosebleed the other day and had to be admitted to the hospital. That kind of stuff. See ya."

The benign, unmodulated way he talked was both puzzling and disconcerting to Janet. The man she had worked for nearly ten years was a stranger. It was her feeling that Father Greer might have been testing himself with the stop at St. Patrick's, but she had gotten no indication as what the result might be.

She asked if people might begin to visit him. He said no.

Father Joseph Payne, his spiritual director, defied that ban, arriving unannounced at St. Mary's rectory two weeks later. He said straightforwardly that "I am the one who needs to see you, Joe, whether or not you want to see me." Father Payne had been distressed that he and Father Greer had not had their final session before the transplant and that he had not been more aggressive in seeing Father Greer—even though his calls, like many others', had not been returned.

Father Payne had made the trip to Charlestown to offer not spiritual solace, but human friendship. He was not there to talk of the state of Father Greer's soul, simply to see if, as one man to another, he might enjoy some companionship. Father Payne asked if they might go to lunch some day. Father Greer said he was not feeling up to it, with enough finality that Father Payne did not pursue it further.

Again Father Greer mentioned the hundred days and his concern that he was not progressing fast enough to prevent "some decisions being made about what to do with me in the future."

Father Payne was about to ask what those "decisions" might be, but the look on Father Greer's face prohibited any further discussion.

9

No, I have not lost my faith. The expression "to lose one's faith," as one might a purse or ring of keys, has always seemed to me rather foolish. . . . Faith is not a thing which one "loses," we merely cease to shape our lives by it.

The first report came from the Service d'Hématologie et d'Immunohématologie, Hôpital Saint-Louis, and the Centre de Transfusion sanguine, Hôpital Trousseau, both in Paris, and the Service de radiothérapie, Institut Gustave Roussy, in Villejuif, France.

The second report, released in the same month, was from the National Conference of Catholic Bishops, in Washington.

The first was cautiously optimistic about Father Greer's disease; the second, decidedly pessimistic about his profession.

A team of French physicians had treated eight multiple myeloma patients with precisely the same regime Father Greer had received: high-dose chemotherapy and total body irradiation followed by an infusion of the patient's own peripheral stem cells. Except for one patient who had died of cerebral bleeding forty days after transplant, the results had been dramatic. Five patients were off therapy and well—two in what the doctors termed "apparent complete remission" and the other three with only "minimal residual disease"—a condition, the doctors noted, that another transplant patient had been living with for seven years. Seven of the eight were still alive, the longest for almost a year and a half.

It was a small sample and the follow-up time was short, but nonetheless the report from France was highly significant. It was the first extended study of a group of myeloma who had received this innovative treatment. All the living patients had regrown the blood cells needed to sustain life, most of them within the first two months posttransplant. "Our results . . . although preliminary, seem encouraging," the French doctors concluded in the classic terms of understatement researchers restrict themselves to on the threshold of a breakthrough.

If the paper from France was greeted with enthusiasm by trans-plant physicians worldwide—as it was at the New England Medical Center—the report from Washington received a corporate groan from American priests. Once again they were the subject of a study; once again the news was discouraging about the state of *their* health.

The survey, commissioned by the United States bishops and intended at first for their use only, painted—or repainted—a picture of which they had certainly been aware. Nonetheless, in both scope and depth it was far more bleak than they had anticipated. So serious were the findings that the bishops had decided to pass them on to American priests without any omissions.

"Although there are present today powerful individual examples of priestly ministry shared in creative and energizing ways which continue the mission and ministry of the church, it is also clear that there exists today a serious and substantial morale problem among priests in general," the report read. "American priesthood is in the season of its mid-life crisis . . ." and ". . . there are a significant number who have settled for a part-time presence to their priesthood. . . . This is particularly true of those in the 45 to 60 age group who are willing to go through the necessary motions but whose hearts and energies are elsewhere."

Directly addressing the shortage of qualified priests, it noted, "Bishops and personnel boards find themselves giving full and total pastoral responsibilities to men who could serve well and happily only in carefully limited capacities." In conclusion, the report said, "We have been struck by the fact that priests' morale today seems particularly fragile, rather easily influenced and, in many ways, a highly sensitive barometer of what is going on in church and society."

Each report exerted a certain pressure upon Father Greer, who week after week returned to the hematology/oncology clinic for transfusions. One was saying he could reasonably expect to get better. The other that—as he was one of that ever-shrinking contingent of qualified, committed priests—he should get back to work as soon as possible.

Ostensibly St. Patrick's had been functioning smoothly during its pastor's absence, but Father Greer knew the undertow of parish life, that a church with eighty-five hundred members could drift along only so long with a caretaker pastor, even as well intentioned a man as Father Greer knew Father Moritz to be. A firm hand was needed at the tiller.

Father Moritz, while an experienced pastor and overwhelmingly liked by the parish staff, was not about to make any major decisions at St. Patrick's. This was understandable enough, considering his time there was supposed to be limited. He was also seventy-two years old and had had some neurological problems lately, a tingling in his arms and fingers for which physicians had yet to find a cause. As she had intimated, Janet Hamilton, the parish secretary, was feeling overburdened. Not only had many of the administrative tasks Father Greer normally handled fallen to her, but there was a sudden spate of maintenance problems—from leaking pipes to the major renovation of the kitchen—and also policy questions such as the videotaping of weddings, a practice which Father Greer had forbidden, but which was now being done. What was she supposed to do? She was only the parish secretary, a woman with responsibilities, yet no real power.

Father Rossi, who had officiated at more of the parish's weddings than any other priest—was scheduled to leave in mid-June, at the height of the marriage season. While Father Mullaney was taking a share of the weddings that came in, he was a man who, by seniority, would soon have his own parish. It was not to be expected that he would approach the work as a curate with the same enthusiasm as Father Rossi, still on his first assignment after ordination.

Parishioners were grumbling—nothing new to Father Greer— but for the time being he was hardly in a position to address their complaints. The missalettes no longer contained the Sunday readings (a change proposed by the parish liturgy committee to encourage worshipers to listen to the word of God and not read it), and a group of parishioners were outraged. The nine o'clock weekday morning Mass had been eliminated, leaving only the eight o'clock, and that irritated another segment of the parish. Along with cards and letters offering prayers and good thoughts for his recovery, Father Greer began to receive irate letters demanding that the changes be rescinded immediately.

Both the parish and Father Greer's body were voicing their metabolic demands. For the moment, neither was having its needs met.

Day 100 passed. Day 110. Day 120. Day 130.

Because his blood counts had improved marginally, Father Greer's visits to the clinic had been reduced to one a week. But this weekly visit—and above all, what it confirmed, that his marrow was not producing well enough to sustain life—was taking its toll on him, a man who had been too intimately linked to the New England Medical Center over the past five months. His blood counts persisted at low levels—hematocrit or red cell count at around 27 (40 to 50 is the normal range), white cell count at 1.6 (normal is between 6 and 10), and platelets, 7,000 (150,000 to 250,000 is normal).

Each Tuesday, Father Greer planned on spending a full day at the center: his 10 A.M. exam by Drs. Shulman and Desforges and the results of his blood counts invariably required him to appear at the blood bank on the eighth floor to receive transfusions of red blood cells and platelets. A special cleansing and irradiation of the blood products, necessary to prevent unwanted antibodies from disturbing his already fragile hematological ecosystem, took a minimum of an hour and a half. As he customarily received two bags of red cells and one of platelets, he did not finish until late in the afternoon.

As for the other six days of the week: Father Greer was feeling generally awful.

He had moved to the Immaculate Conception rectory in Everett, which was closer to the hospital. The pastor, Father Edward Sviokla, was an old friend.

Father Greer found himself in an unabated state of fatigue. He needed an afternoon nap and went to bed exhausted around seven P.M. Although he would be in bed for ten hours, he had difficulty achieving any sustained sleep. He would be awakened in the night by the tug of the lumens he could never comfortably secure to his chest. His joints and muscles ached, his throat was sore. He knew too well the Boston stations that carried all-night talk shows. He woke in the morning choking, his mouth brimming with the gelatinous residue of mucositis. He walked the lonely streets at dawn, his companions the elderly of Everett, equally unable to sleep.

When he said a private Mass in his room, he had to remain seated for most of it and even then periodically rested to recoup his energy and refocus his constantly wandering mind. On his head a modest growth of black peach fuzz was maturing into thicker strands of hair, but vanity was not a concern.

Father Greer was tired of being tired, tired of being sick, tired of not being able to concentrate for more than fifteen minutes, tired of eating chicken or stew or tuna fish that were equally tasteless. Tired of afternoons—once filled with CCD classes, hospital visits, and counseling sessions—that now dragged by. He was tired of living in a rectory where he had no purpose.

Father Greer was tired of the hematological limbo to which he felt himself condemned. The bone marrow transplant had not killed him, but neither had it rewarded him with anything resembling a normal life. He was a man on a medical tether from which he could do nothing to free himself. All he could do was the one thing that had always been the hardest and cruelest punishment for him: nothing.

He had to wait.

And while it was excruciating to spend as much time alone as he did, Father Greer kept the wall around him up, discouraging people from visiting, rejecting most invitations to go for lunch or dinner. "For what?" he would say. "I can't taste anything anyhow; what's the use of going out?"

Father Greer eventually allowed me back into his life—my threatened dismissal in the weeks immediately after his release from the hospital was never mentioned—and I began to take him for his weekly clinic visits. But I quickly realized our relationship had changed. At first, it was difficult for me to sort out how I had come to play a new and curious role in his life. It took a number of trips to the clinic for me to begin to understand.

The occasional visitor to a hematology/oncology clinic, such as that at the New England Medical Center, might feel unsettled at seeing a room filled with people who have serious diseases, many of them with little hope for recovery. As cheery as the staff can be, nothing can disguise the fact that this is a gathering place for the very ill, whose prospects can quickly be assessed from their vacant stares and their looks of unmasked anguish.

For the regular patient who week after week sees the same faces infused with pain or numbed with lassitude, it is a constant reminder of his or her own sickness, the fact that each of them is indeed very, very ill, perhaps a fragile foothold away from the most afflicted or pathetic person in the room. The patients constantly posit mental comparisons. ("I don't look that bad, do I? Did I? Will I?") But then a day comes when a face—pained as it was the last time—is no longer present. Or there is a new face or a new head scalded by radiation, or another body slumped in a wheelchair, another wife or husband or brother or sister vainly trying to look brave as he or she sits beside the person clutching a new clinic card. Such patients are recognizable not only by the newness of their faces, but because they are the ones who, while sitting in the waiting area, talk to the family member or friend who brought them.

Regular patients have long ago used up their supply of words.

Whatever the distance the regular patient might feel between him- or herself and the others in the room, he or she feels weaker just being there, surrounded by so much sickness. There is no protection from such an aura, no mental gymnastic that can be effectively exercised, and for Father Greer there was not even a spiritual weapon that could be summoned to drive the curse from the place.

Father Greer had become a member of an exclusive club, in which membership is never sought and from which resignation is impossible. He, Jackie Forest, John Andrews, Peter Edwards, John Johnson and the two Italian men whose nationality he knew but not their names, all were inextricably linked together. Regular patients know—sometimes correctly and sometimes not—all about each others' state. Whether transfusions are required or a hospitalization has occurred. How many days each of those who has had a marrow or stem cell transplant was in an isolation room. What chemotherapy drugs they take. What the side effects are. Blood counts, appetite, sleeping habits.

Regardless of the type of blood disease or cancer they have—each type having its own range of severity and therefore its different percentages of remission and cure—patients relentlessly compare themselves to the others being treated. It makes no difference to them that great strides have been made in curing certain disorders while others remain uniformly fatal. What does matter is that one patient is about to return to work, another is eating well, another sleeping through the night.

And that they themselves are or are not.

These days it was John Andrews, a man Father Greer rarely saw during his Tuesday appointments, who was the talk of the clinic. His marrow transplant, received from his brother, had engrafted quickly at the Hutchinson Center in Seattle, and five weeks later he had gone back to work. It was emblematic of the spate of false or partial information that passed for fact at the clinic that no one was aware that Andrews, almost immediately after the transplant, began to show signs that the myeloma had returned.

As the patients sat in the clinic, the blood bank, the X-ray department—there was always ample opportunity to wait—they heard from one another the latest miracle cure and immediately started to imagine whether it might work for them: a doctor in Greece whose serum selectively attacked the coating of cancer cells; interferon; the charismatic healing priest, Father D'Orio; a new high-fiber diet; vitamin E; interleukin-2. Hokum, faith, and high medical science mingled indiscriminately, stirred in some by hope, in others by desperation.

And Father Greer, never one to subscribe to the surfeit of miracles in everyday life, listened and nodded as each was propounded, neither dismissing the apparently foolish nor subscribing to what seemed medically sound.

Poor as he was feeling physically and despite the additional debilitation he was suffering from the onslaughts of his recurring and unpredictable depression, Father Greer, to my surprise, was not one to wear a long face once he was in the clinic or at the blood bank receiving a transfusion. At first I had thought it was just my imagination, but then, as I noted it week after week, I could see that something inside him changed when he walked through that door to face those charged with restoring him to health.

He mentioned his fatigue and lack of ability to taste in response to his doctors' questions, but he did not unduly complain. "Felt better, felt better, believe me," he would say. If they asked him if he had visited his home in New Hampshire, he would inquire about their weekend skiing trip or vacation to the Caribbean. Up in the blood bank, chatting with Carol or Lisa or Allen as the needed blood cells flowed from a suspended plastic bag into his catheter, he was always ready with a pithy remark about "blood bank time" (his transfusions inevitably started late and ended beyond the promised time of completion) or whatever local or national scandal, aberration, or foolishness was dominating the news.

The blood bank personnel were delighted with his peppy responses; there had been so many weeks just after the transplant when he would barely talk to them. The old Father Greer was back, they felt; his counts might be lagging, but he was getting better.

When Father Greer paid a visit to Proger 6 North one week in between his examination and transfusion, he was given a hero's homecoming. He was beaming. Female nurses who had once handled him with rubber gloves and talked through paper masks threw their arms around him and kissed his cheek. Danny McClellan lifted Father Greer's terry-cloth golf cap and tousled the sparse growth. He had returned—as so few of their patients who had survived a transplant do—and he was ruddy and smiling and he remembered their names and told Danny that his Celtics tickets were assured; he just wanted to make sure Larry Bird was back in the lineup before he got them.

They told him how good he looked and he replied, "Better get my marrow to be looking good, too," as if it were merely a cosmetic concern like the regrowth of his hair.

But it was another Father Greer I saw during our trips to and from the clinic, in the hours over coffee in the cafeteria waiting for his blood to be readied.

Father Greer had just finished reading a biography of Thomas Merton, the Trappist monk and writer who was the subject of a television documentary and book I had done, and he dismissed Merton coldly as "a wanderer who didn't know who he was or what he wanted. Ended up a Buddhist, didn't he?"

In the course of a conversation I casually mentioned a new book I was reading, Paul Johnson's *A History of the Jews*, and told Father

Greer how many things I was learning from it, including the theory that God had offered his pact ("You will be my people and I will be your God") to a number of the wandering tribes of the day, but that only the Israelites had accepted it. I underscored that it was only a theory forwarded in the book, but Father Greer lashed out at me for even mentioning it, saying categorically that "Everyone knows there was a chosen people, *one specific* chosen people."

When he got into the car one morning, I asked how he was feeling, and he snapped: "Asking me how I'm feeling is like saying, 'We'll have lunch sometime,' or 'I'll get back to you on that.' Ask me how is my cancer; that's the proper question." And on another Tuesday, after not seeing him for two weeks, I asked how his blood counts were. He replied in a clipped tone, "I know exactly what they are before I go in. I know what I feel like, the counts only confirm what I feel like."

I had always enjoyed his ready and self-deprecating wit, and I realized that the words in these retorts were not unlike those he might have used months before. But something had changed. There was a bitterness in his voice, a caustic quality of which I had not thought him capable.

As we spent hours together, I struggled to come up with topics of conversation that would not anger him, but I failed miserably. As his hair grew out, I said in a congratulatory voice that he'd need a haircut soon. "I'll wait until spring. Want me to catch a cold?" I asked if he could taste anything, even the Manhattans he and I had once enjoyed in our evenings together. "Asking me about taste is like asking me what color I see. I'm color-blind. Remember?" He said something about the state Capitol building as we walked along Boston Common one morning, and I casually remarked I had never noticed the gold-domed building, which, I could now see, dominated the area.

"You really don't know much about Boston, do you?"

Missing badly on temporal issues, I stumbled into the spiritual. I asked him one day what illness teaches a person. I tried to be specific, as he had bade me to do when I dealt in generalities. I used the word "enrich." "Enrich me? What are you talking about? I'm dealing with an illness, myself. Enrichment is dealing with other people."

Where was the colloquial, congenial man I had seen in the examining room and the blood bank? How could he be so friendly in those places, but so tough on me? I began to feel like the wife of the wonderfully warm and witty cocktail party host who, once all the guests leave, routinely finds herself the target of a tirade or cutting verbal abuse.

It took awhile, but finally I thought I understood.

Father Greer was living as a guest in a rectory and surely must have felt he had outstayed his welcome. He had no responsibilities in his home parish and little contact with it, and was in no position to tell the man who was there covering for him when he would be relieved. When the occasional friend came to call or to take him to another tasteless lunch or dinner, what could he say? How could he explain or act out the impotence he felt—his malaise, his frustration, his pain, his fear?

He had avoided seeing his spiritual director, Father Payne. As for his priest friends, if the lack of candor and real intimacy I had witnessed when he was with them before the transplant was any indication, I doubted Father Greer was being particularly forthcoming with them about his current experiences.

I don't mean to overstate my role in his life. I never felt I was all that important to Father Greer; whether I spent time with him or wrote about him was irrelevant to him. But I was somebody he had been with a lot over the previous two years, somebody who didn't fit into the category of those either treating him or served by him. And, I wasn't really a friend. Of course there was some sort of bond, but I never presumed upon it, and I felt that as fond as I was of him, the relationship was somehow impersonal. He never initiated a phone call to me for any reason.

Perhaps it was my "indeterminate" status that made me the one person on whom he could readily take out his innermost frustration. He knew that as insufferable as he was toward me, I would not go away.

In some small way, and masked by his icy and unkind remarks, I was seeing that deepest side of him, his rage at the limbo in which he was being forced to live, at his interminable malaise, his lack of mental acuity. When I finally began to understand why he was acting as he did toward me, I found (putting my ego aside, as well as the compassion I felt for what he was going through) it frightened me.

For inside, Father Greer was not healing, only growing more morose. It was a repeat of what had happened after the transplant when, even as his doctors maintained that his recovery was proceeding on schedule, Father Greer refused to allow himself to believe he would improve. And as the days passed, the hope of a full recovery of his bone marrow became slimmer. Father Greer had constantly maintained he was not afraid to die. Now the question was: Was he equally unafraid to live if it meant living in this reduced state? He had wanted a miracle—who could blame him?—and it had not happened.

Father Greer's doctors watched his counts closely, and they were puzzled. Why was his marrow producing with such limited results? He had started to engraft in almost record time but then hit a plateau he could not get beyond. Had the stem cells they had infused been permanently damaged in their regenerative capabilities by the extensive chemotherapy he had undergone? While the drugs had twice put the myeloma into remission or had kept it at an acceptable level as the preparations for the transplant proceeded, had they rendered sterile the cells he needed to sustain life? Or were there simply not enough of them? Had the myeloma itself so damaged the structural microenvironment of his bone marrow—the delicate honeycomb within which blood cells are produced—as to preclude sustained regrowth?

Was the problem at the beginning of the cycle—were insufficient numbers of new stem cells being produced in Father Greer's marrow to begin the necessary chain reaction—or was it at the end, that is, were antibodies for some unknown reason destroying his healthy red and white blood cells and his platelets as soon as he produced them?

Drs. Desforges, Shulman, Miller, and Hillyer knew what questions to pose, but they had no answers. Neither did anyone else. The number of multiple myeloma cases that had been treated with transplants was so tiny, the follow-up time so short, that no one could point with any certainty to the cause of Father Greer's state—called an "incomplete recovery"—or postulate his chances for a complete recovery.

All the New England Medical Center team could say with certainty was the obvious: their patient was alive. And by this time, had the transplant not been performed and the second round of chemotherapy eventually proven ineffective, as it often does—he might have been dead. Father Greer had had no serious infections since the herpes, though his white cell count was low. He had not had any bleeding that could not be controlled, although his platelets were below the acceptable level. And the continuing protein electrophoresis tests showed no sign whatsoever that the myeloma had returned.

The doctors could reassure themselves with the thought that here was a man who was living on borrowed time, and most likely it was their efforts that had extended his life. But of course, that was not enough. They did not want only that their medical procedure succeed; to them Father Greer was a patient they uniformly admired—and yes, by now, loved.

"I guess his feistiness is the most appealing thing about him," said Dr. Hillyer. "I've taken care of other priests, and they would always say something like 'If God tells me it's time, I'll go.' Father Greer looked up at me when I was injecting the second batch of stem cells and said, 'This better work, my friend.' This man in no way wants to die."

Dr. Shulman, who during her short medical career had already seen her share of patients slip away, was constantly aware of the parallels between Father Greer and her own father. "If anything happened to Father Greer, everybody up here would mourn, as they do for every patient they lose. For me it would be more than that."

Along with the doctors' concern about the lack of Father Greer's progress and a certain surprise at the seemingly positive face he was presenting, there was a consensus that Father Greer was, in Dr. Desforges's words, "Dragging his heels a bit." They sensed that something was holding him back, that he could and should begin to be thinking about doing some limited parish work. He had, Rebecca Shulman said, "Gotten used to the role of being a patient. It often happens with a long illness."

But despite their intuition that he could do more, they were agreed that none of them had gone through what he had and none was really in a position to know his actual capacities.

Father Greer was not one to question or blame them or ask them for a miraculous cure, as many of their patients do. He never contacted them outside his normal appointments. Even the night he had had the nosebleed, he had waited until the blood had saturated his pillow before he called. Rarely during examinations did he seem vulnerable or defenseless before them.

Rarely. But there were glimpses registered by Dr. Desforges, seasoned clinician that she was, that indicated that Father Greer was not revealing everything going on inside him.

One morning, Dr. Desforges completed her examination of Father Greer and moved to another patient in the room, whose bed was sectioned off by curtains. That examination over, she passed Father Greer, who had just finished dressing and was about to leave. Uncharacteristically, he blurted out a question.

"When is it going to happen?"

Before she could make any reply, he said, "Every time I ask myself that, I say to myself: Why did I ask that? As we say in philosophy, it's not a valid question. I know. You don't know. I don't know. Nobody . . ." his voice trailed off.

10

But then God helped me. Suddenly I could feel a tear on my cheek, a single tear, as we see them on the faces of the dying, at the furthest limit of their griefs.

Within a period of forty-eight hours in early March, Father Greer sent a series of mixed signals. He told Dr. Miller he was "feeling pretty good." He called Janet the parish secretary to check in, but when asked when he might return to St. Patrick's, informed her, "It's a matter of *if* I come back." He told Dr. Desforges that he would concelebrate Mass publicly on Holy Thursday. He angrily berated me for sending him what I thought was an insightful article.

I tried to decipher these contradictory communications but could not. But something was happening in the life of Father Joseph Greer.

This trail of messages had begun with a chance meeting with Dr. Kenneth Miller, whom Father Greer did not normally see on his weekly visits. Dr. Miller, who was almost running through the hematology/oncology waiting room on his way from the parking garage to his office, stopped and asked how the priest was doing. Father Greer's response was immediate, and unlike what might have been expected from the lifeless man with whom I had just spent the past two hours, energetic and positive. "But the marrow doesn't understand what's needed here, does it?" Father Greer added, as if a workman had hung a door the wrong way and would have to come back to put the job right.

"Inscrutable, that's all I can say," Dr. Miller responded. "Has an agenda of its own. But we're so pleased with your recovery. You're doing so good otherwise."

"With the accent on otherwise, right? Let's talk to whoever's in charge of these counts and get them moving." They laughed together.

The phone call to Janet Hamilton had been made during a week when all hell was breaking loose at St. Patrick's. The chancery had discovered another problem with the cemetery bids, a new leak in the rectory sprinkler system had ruined a ceiling, grumbling parishioners were beginning to defect to neighboring parishes over the new missalettes and Mass times, and Leonard Morse Hospital had complained that one of the curates had been missing his rounds.

Janet poured out her frustration in an uninterrupted monologue and ended with, "Listen, buddy, when the hell are you getting back here, anyhow?"

It was then that Father Greer emphasized that the question was "if" not "when," and he was soon off the phone, having offered no advice on what to do.

Dr. Desforges smiled broadly as she stood before her patient, her blue eyes magnified and gleaming behind her thick glasses as she learned of the Mass he would participate in.

"Holy Thursday? Wonderful. Now that will be a cause for celebration, won't it?"

"I figure if I'm tired, or getting wobbly, I can just walk off the altar; nobody will know the difference," the priest told her.

"It sounds just right to me," she said. "Dr. Shulman?"

"I concur absolutely," she said, her hand on Father Greer's arm. "It's time."

After his appointment, as we rode back to Everett, I mentioned that he must be feeling better. I told him how happy that made me. There was no response. I stumbled on, wanting somehow to fill in the uneasy stillness that had descended upon the car. "That piece on prayer in *Commonweal* I sent you; pretty nicely put, I thought. Made sense."

Silence.

"At least to me. Prayer isn't exactly the easiest subject to write about. I think he did a pretty good job of—"

"It's in the hands of God, not man," he cut me off, irritation in his voice. "Not much to it; read it all before. Man trying to figure out what God is thinking. God thinking? Man, puny man, tries to figure things out. It brought God down to our level. What kind of foolishness is that? What kind of God would that be? Nobody takes the place of God. Foolish!"

I mumbled something in response and asked if he hoped to play golf in Florida.

He left for a ten-day vacation at a friend's condominium near Naples, Florida, and his absence gave me time to think further about the two Father Greers I was encountering. I found myself coming back time and again to Dr. Desforges's words just before the transplant: that transplant patients rarely go back to doing what they did before the procedure. The trauma of the transplant, the frightening period when marrow either engrafts or doesn't, the haunting days in isolation, the continuing sickness and weariness all conspire to disorient even the most stable personality. Dr. Desforges had allowed during that conversation that Father Greer, even though he obviously relished his work, would have to go through a period where he sorted out whether he really wanted to return to it.

There was a battle being waged within the man, that much was obvious. It was not whether or not he would remain a priest and function as one, but rather if he could—as he had articulated so many times—truly accept the burden of his illness. Lay it down and go on. It is the kind of acceptance he had always talked about, the grace of forgiveness of self, regardless of circumstances.

He had known deep inner conflict before. At some point after he had violated his vow of chastity, he had decided he could no longer go on sinning and had to confront his sinfulness if he could ever expect to leave it behind. He had had to look into the murky corners of his shadow side and face what he saw there; he had had to admit that was part of him too. After priests had begun to leave in the freedom of the post–Vatican II era and he wondered why he himself was staying, he had come to the realization that while the priesthood he had signed on for was not the priesthood he would be living, he could not have any other life and be satisfied with it. Faced with his own narrow views of church law and human failings, he had eventually admitted that it was he and his majestic Mother Church who had been too harsh, too righteous, too loveless—and had to change.

Father Greer was again being summoned to an honesty that was easy to articulate but so difficult to live out.

He could perform in the clinic, but then he lay awake through dark nights of the soul. He pushed himself to walk further and read longer, but his body and mind scoffed at his will. He was realizing that if he were to go back to the life of a priest in a huge parish, it would not be as a man who has been miraculously cured and was again whole.

He would come back a man who was himself in continuing and obvious need.

Father Greer had been humbled by his own failings and had become a better, more compassionate priest because of them. But the inner deficiencies had not shown. Now there was no way of hiding.

Father Greer, wearing the white stole of Holy Thursday, which symbolizes the joy and festivity of this pivotal day of the church year, looked calm, rested, and well as he stood off to one side of the altar under the soaring, vaulted arches of Immaculate Conception Church of Everett. Father Joseph O'Sullivan, the curate, and a visiting priest on the opposite side of the altar, were also concelebrating the evening Mass. Of the three, Father Greer, with a healthy tan on his face from his Florida vacation, looked the most fit. The pastor, Father Edward Sviokla, Father Greer's longtime friend who had provided him with a home the past few months, was the principal celebrant. At the Gospel, Father Sviokla, a huge man, hovered like a enormous shrouded eagle over the opened Bible before him and leaned out from the pulpit as he read the powerful words of the thirteenth chapter of John in a resonant baritone voice: "Jesus realized that the hour had come . . ."

It was chilly and damp in the cavernous church; only a token of heat had been offered up before the service, and the radiators were now still and cold.

". . . for him to pass from this world to the Father . . ."

I watched Father Greer, but there was no movement on his face. He was listening, as I was, but what were these words meaning to him as he sat there on the altar for the first time in six months?

". . . He had loved his own in the world and would show his love for them to the end . . ."

The solemn pageantry of Holy Thursday continued, as the final hours of Christ's life were reenacted. His time was limited, and in parting He took the place of a servant and washed the feet of his apostles, giving them an example to follow, and then provided food for their journey. Taking bread and then wine, He transformed these staples of their meal into His body and blood.

In the course of the Mass, Father Sviokla knelt to wash the feet of some of his parishioners. At the Consecration, he intoned Christ's words:

"This is my body which will be given up for you. . . . This is my blood . . ."

Had Father Greer consciously chosen this night? It was all about commitment to the priesthood, exactly what he was facing. So many words were so poignant; how did they strike him? After Mass I hurried back to the Immaculate Conception rectory to await him.

As we sat in the rectory parlor and I could see him up close, he once more looked very tired. He seemed at times to miss a breath and then had to draw the next with even more intent. His forehead was glossy with perspiration. He tugged at the Roman collar he was wearing and I asked, after all these months, if it still fit.

He smiled and nodded, understanding the literal and metaphorical implications. "Getting a little jowly, but I can still get the thing on."

I asked about the service.

"It was good to be up there with priests again," he said. "To feel the real Presence. I felt a little weak there once, but after I was up on the altar for the Consecration, I was able to wipe it out of my mind and I lost the tiredness."

The words?

"Sort of tough to have the words pop out at you after you've been saying them for almost thirty-one years."

Any words at all that had struck him?

"No, not really."

The room was silent and I waited, for often Father Greer follows a dismissal with an insight. This time there was none.

"A very important night for you, isn't it?" I asked.

"Yes. Sort of like spring training. To see if I can really hit the ball again."

"You seem in better spirits; has anything changed? Maybe it was Florida."

"Changed?"

I was censoring my comments, but they still came out jumbled and foolish. "Something is different . . . well, I just thought you were a little rough on me during the past couple months. Seems I couldn't say anything right. You bit my head off more than once."

He looked at me blankly. I sensed he was going back in time to recall even one such incident. He could not.

"So where do you think the change came about? Something is different; I don't know what it is, but it's different. What about Florida?"

He looked at me blankly again. He was thinking.

"My first golf of the year. I hit eighty-seven down there. My usual for this time of the year."

"I see."

Father Greer shifted uneasily in his chair. He looked down at his watch, and I was ready to be told to go.

"Back a ways you asked me . . ." he said slowly. A thought had flickered into consciousness, and in his fatigue he was at once struggling to keep hold of it and to find the words to express it. "You asked what I learned from the illness. I learned that everybody has things going on inside that no one has the least idea about . . .

"I learned not to be so quick to judge. I can identify with weakness now; I lost faith. I understand how people can do it. And when you're feeling so low, nothing seems to matter; your chin is on your chest. You're not hopeful, and you can't be helpful to anybody.

"I look at the people I see in clinic—one of the Italian guys used to weigh 220; he's down to 110 with colon cancer and they can't do a thing for him. I saw three deaths in the paper last week from myeloma. I can't complain. I'm beginning to taste food, if I put a lot of salt on it. I can read for twenty minutes at a stretch. I know what a struggle it's been just to get to ground zero.

"And the weather looks like it finally's getting warmer. The worst of winter is over. Now get out of here so I can get to bed."

On Easter Sunday Father Greer said the afternoon Mass at Immaculate Conception. He was alone on the altar for the first time since he had entered the hospital over six months before. Immediately following the Mass, he stripped off his clothes, which were drenched with perspiration, took a shower, and went to bed.

Three years before, on Easter Sunday, he had said Mass at Leonard Morse sitting up in a wheelchair that had been brought into the chapel. Three years, the statistical average life span from diagnosis to death for a multiple myeloma patient.

Father Greer had passed that point on Dr. Desforges's chart, the line of demarcation between the living and the dead.

On the trees along East Central Street in front of St. Patrick's the static branches of winter began to swell. There were no blossoms yet, no readily visible life upon them, but the signs were unmistakable. Easter, which had come early this year, had passed. Once again, spring's life had triumphed over winter's death.

Janet Hamilton, Father Joseph Payne, and Christina Wilhelm saw equally portentous signs of another kind on a Monday morning in April, some two weeks after Easter. Others in Father Greer's wide circle of friends, fellow priests, employees, and parishioners past and present may have seen additional indications, but they had found no way of keeping one another abreast of the state of the man for whom they had been so fervently hoping and praying since the October days when the leaves had fallen from the trees and life was systematically eliminated from his body.

Father Payne saw him first that Monday morning when Father Greer detoured to the priory in Dover on his way from Everett to Natick. Although Father Payne had called him the week before and Father Greer had not seemed eager to meet, it was Father Greer who had proposed this visit. Father Greer arrived, as Father Payne would tell me later, "in play clothes, for the first time in anything other than clerics," and for a while they traded shop talk (the priory was being sued over its use of the enneagram in workshops; what to do about St. Patrick's loss of Father Rossi, with no replacement in sight) before they went to the private room where they usually had their session. When they got there, Father Payne noted—as a retreat master and spiritual director, a practiced and astute observer of human nuance—that Father Greer proceeded not to the stiff-backed chair near the small end table, but rather to a comfortable overstuffed chair near the window.

Father Payne did not take his usual chair across the room from Father Greer, but instead sat on a sofa. They spent their usual hour together, with far more time spent on catching up on each other's lives—and the jumbled lives of their respective institutions—than on any deep, pressing issue on the mind of the spiritual directee.

Christina Wilhelm had been the target of parish criticism since the first missalette had appeared without the Sunday readings, Father Greer related to Father Payne. Accused of overstepping her authority as liturgical director, of violating church law, and of infringing on worshipers' rights, she too had heard of parishioners who were indignantly going to St. Linus and Sacred Heart, the two other Natick Catholic churches. She had thought the change, so small, would hardly be noticed. She had been crushed by the response. The two priests smiled at the loyalty of the Catholic parishioner.

Christina Wilhelm was standing in the parish office when Father Greer entered through the back door, having parked his car at the rear of the church. The look on her face bespoke her distress.

"Don't worry about it, Christina," Father Greer said, even before she could utter a word. "Wait till I hit them with the renovation of the upper church. That'll get them off your back and they'll put the heat on me—" He hesitated. She looked at him, a grin beginning to arch her cheeks.

"—again," he added. "Two years it'll take and a half million bucks. You'll be small potatoes."

Once Mrs. Wilhelm had left, Father Greer took one of his own concerns to Janet.

"The pigeon droppings on the canopy over the elevator," he said, his expression not dissimilar from the one he had presented in the worst days of nausea after the transplant. "Can't we do something about that?"

"The custodian was waiting for better weather so—" Janet began.

"The fire department. Wait a minute! I bet they could get at it real easy. What's that number?" He dialed. "Is the chief there? Father Greer at St. Patrick's."

His call completed, Father Greer went upstairs to his room to get his swimming trunks, goggles, and swim cap.

. . .

The next day in the hematology/oncology clinic, Father Greer's hematocrit and platelet counts were sufficiently high for him not to need a transfusion. He called Janet at noon from Immaculate Conception, and matching the origin of the call and the hour she quickly deduced the significance.

"You want to know why you didn't need a transfusion today, buddy?" she said.

"Why?"

"Because yesterday you made some Father Greer calls, that's why. Now, when are you coming back?"

This time he had an answer.

As Father Greer lay on the examining table during his next appointment at the hematology/oncology clinic, awaiting the arrival of Drs. Shulman and Desforges with the blood counts, he commented to the nurse how it had taken three days to be tested and transfused in Florida and that he would never again accuse the staff on the eighth floor of working on "blood bank time."

"Now, there's a familiar voice!"

Father Greer looked at the curtain a few feet to his left. "Now, who would that be calling out to me?"

The nurse pulled back the curtain to reveal a thin, attractive woman in her early twenties with short curly hair a radiant shade of auburn.

"Could this be Jackie Forest?" he said. "Why, you might have gained a half a pound. Now, did I actually see you in the hospital or just hear about your birdlike appetite? Brain wasn't exactly on all its cylinders those days."

"Actually gained three last week," she grinned. "And you got your hair back. Sure, you saw me; I saw you. My hair came back even curlier. And look at the color. Couldn't even get this out of a bottle. You look great, Father Greer."

"Tell my marrow how great I look. How's the appetite? Eating better? How's the strength? I never thought I'd need a nap every afternoon. Transfusions? Unfortunately, I'm still one of their best customers upstairs."

"No transfusions, and the appetite's a little better. At least I'm keeping it down. No naps, but I sleep until eleven in the morning. You look just great!"

"I can't shift out of neutral. Didn't need any reds or platelets last week, but I've had these false starts before."

"You look *great*," she said, "even—even if you are a priest!"

Three hours later, Father Greer was again reclining. This time his face had that frightening stillness of a man whose hopes had again been dashed. When Dr. Desforges had said he would need two units of red blood cells, Father Greer had met the news with a resigned nod of his head.

She had asked how he was feeling. And Father Greer had responded with the date of his first Mass back at St. Patrick's.

"I'll take it slow; see how it goes. I know I'm at ground zero and I can't rush it. If I have the stamina, I'll go back on weekends and build up. Hopefully, by September I can go back full time."

Dr. Desforges looked over at Dr. Shulman. "We concur, don't we, Rebecca, that that is an excellent plan."

"We do," the younger doctor said, a huge and uncharacteristically girlish grin on her face.

But for now he was again on the eighth floor in the blood bank, the first unit of red cells hanging above him on an IV pole. It was a busy day for Carol and Lisa. Allen was on vacation and both pheresis rooms were occupied, each with two patients. All three of the couches were in use: Father Greer on the far left, next to him a middle-aged black woman here for the first time and an older, gaunt man who Father Greer had seen before but did not know. A family—father, mother, and daughter—occupied the small waiting area at the center of the blood bank area. Their conversation was low and solemn but continuous. They, too, were new to the medical center.

The first unit of blood above Father Greer's head was almost spent when a young man joined the family.

Soon after, a young woman was wheeled out of one of the pheresis rooms. Her face was so pale that even her faint, thin eyebrows stood out. The back of her hair was smashed against her skull from too much time on a pillow. The part cruelly revealed prematurely grey strands at the roots.

"Hey, that wasn't so bad, now was it? What a trooper," said the young man, obviously her husband.

"You look great; you'll be up and at 'em in no time," said her father.

"Interleukin. Where did I read about that? *Reader's Digest*, wasn't it? Miracle drug of our time, they call it." Her younger sister smoothed out her hair as she talked to her.

"We're seeing right now if we can bring you home; if you feel up to it, that is," said her mother.

"Oh, I'd like that," she said weakly, forcing a smile. "Yes."

Across the room, Father Greer was watching them with a look I had never seen before from him. His face still retained a certain hardness, even sullenness, but there was another distinct quality in his expression. Unblinking, he stared at them, his eyes filled with an aching so visceral it almost seemed to emit a low moan. He looked as though he might cry. It went beyond the bloodhound's sadness I had noted almost from the start. That had been profound. This was informed.

As we walked out of the hospital later that afternoon, we passed through the third-floor waiting area in The Floating, the pediatric section. A baby cried out, whether from fear or pain or hunger it was impossible to discern. Father Greer never looked to the right or left when he went through this part of the hospital.

We reached the car in the garage.

"The fools," he said bluntly, his voice so bitter I was reluctant to respond or ask to whom he was referring.

"They think they're helping her with all that pep talk. They don't know what she's going through. Interleukin. Experimental. Last resort. They don't know how sick she feels. Trying to make her laugh."

The voice was so unfeeling, so angry. But the eyes I saw in the rearview mirror as we pulled out of the garage were the same as those I had seen in the blood bank as he looked at that frail, sick young woman.

And I realized how inadequate words are to explain what is held in the heart of a person who has truly known pain, who has faced the end of his mortal life.

II

Our Lord seems to smile. Our Lord often smiles. He says to us: "Don't take all these things too seriously."

Late on a Saturday morning, Father Greer pulls off East Central Street and drives into the virtually empty parking lot behind St. Patrick's Church. The lot is freshly paved and newly marked; glistening aluminum bumpers stand in neat rows. The MBTA has finally delivered. It is a clear, sunny late April day, somewhat cool because of a stiff wind from the north that whips at the American flag flying in front of the rectory. The rectory, with its new gutters and white aluminum siding, shimmers in the brilliant sunshine. The church is its ruddy, chapped self but with a new roof of evenly set tiles looks ready to weather many more decades. The awning over the elevator at the side of the church is still streaked with pigeon droppings.

On the ground across the street from the church, below the window of Father Greer's room (someone has hung a "Welcome Back" sign in it) grey, tattered plastic flaps in the breeze, partially covering the area found to contain leakage from an old oil tank. A few twisted I beams lie rusting in a heap. There is a pool of brownish stagnant water at the low spot of the vacant lot, which is now encircled by a cyclone fence. Mr. Andrew Lane's real estate development company has filed for bankruptcy, and the square block is up for sale.

It is the weekend of the fifth Sunday after Easter, a little over a month after the target date Father Greer had set for his return. When he awoke this morning and swung his legs out of bed, they felt leaden. His back was aching. But by the time he got into his car for the twenty-five-minute ride over from Everett, Father Greer had put those infirmities aside.

Father Greer takes a nap after lunch and arrives in the upper church sacristy forty-five minutes before the afternoon Mass is scheduled to begin, allowing himself double his usual time for preparation. He has trouble finding the right switches for the lights in the sanctuary, peering at the numbers through the bifocals he now needs—a by-product of the radiation—and finally takes the glasses off and puts his head inside the panel box. He makes trip after trip to the sanctuary to light the candles, set up the chalice and paten and missal, check the public address system. It is obvious he is both nervous and a bit unsure of how things work here.

In the sacristy the lector, looking for the right words for the occasion, falls back on repeating "We've been thinking about you." Ann Garvey, serving as the extraordinary minister of the Eucharist, tries to give him a welcoming hug; Father Greer backs away from it, patting the site of his Infusaport, a single-line catheter that re- placed the three-lumen Hickman. "Started bleeding the other night; couldn't stop it," he says.

At four o'clock, Jay Perreault, the cantor, offers the congrega- tion—some five to six hundred people, a normal Saturday afternoon gathering—a greeting and enthusiastically adds, "I don't know about you, but it's *wonderful* to have our pastor back with us today."

The applause is immediate and sustained. From the back of the church, Father Greer, the lector, the extraordinary minister, and an altar boy carrying before him a crucifix mounted on a tall staff begin the procession toward the main altar.

The altar boy, new to his job, circles aimlessly about in the sanctuary, not knowing where to rest his burden. Father Greer guides the boy over to the left side and a stand, returns to the center of the sanctuary, and walks up to the microphone. The opening hymn has ended. The church is silent. A number of women have taken out handkerchiefs and are dabbing at their eyes.

"In the Name of the Father and the Son and the Holy Spirit," he begins. "The Lord be with you."

"And also with you," the response is returned. Throats are cleared.

The Mass goes along smoothly, and finally it is time for the Gospel; Father Greer steps into the pulpit. Towering over him is a huge rough-hewn wooden cross, a white cloth draped over the cross beam. It is the symbol of the Christ crucified, who shed his burial cloth and rose from the dead. It is a shroud in size and shape not unlike those in which Father Greer was wrapped when he was taken for total body irradiation.

The Gospel passage is taken from verses near the end of the thirteenth chapter of John.

The words and the voice that delivers them are at once familiar but today infused with new meaning.

> "My children, I am not to be with you much longer.
> "I give you a new commandment:
> "Love one another.
> "Such as my love has been for you,
> "So must your love be for each other."

The Gospel over, Father Greer takes off his glasses and looks out over the seated congregation. He pauses, either collecting his thoughts or savoring what he sees.

"Been a long time," he begins. "Seven months." He nods as if amazed by the number. "A lot of those days were lonely and hurting for me . . . sometimes crying . . . sometimes laughing . . . but I can't tell you how nice it is to come back and see all your faces today. It was no picnic, this transplant, but I'm lucky to have had the chance to go through it. Without it, I would have had one year to live. Now I can give you ten or fifteen more years; not a bad bargain, I think . . ."

His diction is not as crisp as they might have remembered from the autumn; was it the result of the assaults his body had endured; the mucositis? Or was it simply emotion that inhabited his throat? His words go out over the congregation in waves of varying intelligibility. But this is not a tightly reasoned argument that needs to be precisely articulated to be understood.

"I can't put into words what you did for me. It was your prayers and notes and cards and calls that carried me through. Without you I would not have made it. My people did not forget me. Do you know how important that is? The whole process was a good lesson in humility for Father Greer. That St. Patrick's went on before me, went on with me, went on without me.

"I looked like Yul Brynner there for a while. And the memory isn't what it used to be, so I might not remember all your names right away, so please forgive me and give me a little time. There is no cancer in my system, thank God, but the old bone marrow is not exactly clicking in like it should. My white blood cell count is one-point-three—yours is about five—my reds are low, and I'm not making platelets as I should, so I'm open to infection and to bleeding and I run out of gas pretty easily. Where I used to jog eight miles, I now take a walk and the old ladies pass me by. 'I don't know about this marrow of mine,' I was telling my lady Jewish doctor the other day. 'I'm probably getting Protestant transfusions. This ecumenism thing can go too far; just not working here!' "

He pauses until the laughter subsides.

"I want to come back on weekends and see how I do, and if I do okay, I'll come back full time as your pastor in September. But let's take it one step at a time. As you know, being a pastor of a parish this size is—well, quite—trying, shall we say? But, more important, I want you all to know without you I wouldn't be here. You loved me. Now that's enough about me.

"This Gospel is all about love, and how do we love? We can love in the easiest, most straightforward way just by not being critical of each other. Everyone needs support—the person with AIDS, the prisoner, the nonchurchgoer. You. Me. It's what makes it possible for all of us to go on . . ."

Father Greer had wanted to keep his personal remarks shorter and to spend more time on the meaning of the day's Gospel. But he was not able to carry out his plan. After he finished talking about himself, he had but five minutes left of the twelve or so he allows himself. He used the time remaining to address his key point obliquely, as is his style, calling the congregation to account for the conflict within the parish he had heard of during the months away, caused by the missalettes and the new daily Mass times.

"He loves us—with no questions asked. Why are we so stingy

with our love and ready with our criticism of others? We're all
guilty, my friends, all of us."

Father Greer returns to the altar and hesitates for a moment.
Beneath the white polyester alb, his undershirt is soaked through.
He takes a deep breath and turns to his right to receive the cruets
containing wine and water. But the new altar boy has forgotten to
bring the chalice from the small table at the edge of the sanctuary.
So priest and altar boy make the short pilgrimage together to retrieve
the chalice and paten made of Irish crystal, a gift from County
Mayo.

At Mass's end the applause with which the St. Patrick's parishioners greeted Father Greer is repeated even louder. In the vestibule
he shakes hands with all those who present themselves at the door
leading out to East Central Street. He realizes that each hand he
takes—like each hand or mouth on which he had minutes before
placed a Communion Host—is a little island swarming with the
bacteria that still pose a threat.

A few of the women, disregarding his preference, nature, and
white blood cell count, hug him, pressing their cheeks to his, which
are by now flushed and damp. One woman presents him with a
long-stemmed rose.

Before supper there is time for a Manhattan—with plenty of ice—
and a few minutes of a televised golf tournament. The bell for
dinner sounds on the first floor. Only two places would have been
set had I not been there. The other priests are all officiating at
weddings: Father Moritz, the interim pastor, is in Needham, Father
Mullaney is in the upper church, and Father Rossi is in Colorado,
combining a vacation and officiating at the marriage of a friend.

On the dining room table the meal is already set out: asparagus
stalks lie long and limp in a serving dish of the best china, the beans
look equally overcooked, but the rich brown gravy, the smooth,
whipped potatoes, and the finely cut slices of roast prime rib of beef
are right from Dolly's heart, as is the lemon meringue pie that sits
in the kitchen.

As talk around this table is wont to do, it skirts personal trauma
and spiritual darkness and quickly gravitates to the basic realities of
running a parish, of being a priest these days.

A structural engineer commissioned by the archdiocese has pronounced the roof on the school building—long Father Greer's albatross—inadequate; a completely new one is needed. "They want it done, let them come up with the bucks," Father Greer says with more amusement than anger. Weekly attendance is down—Father Greer estimates he is lucky if 20 percent of the Catholics in the parish are now attending Mass. Two more priests have died in the past week, one a few years younger than Father Greer. There are now 904 active priests in the Boston archdiocese. As a favor to some old friends, Father Greer married a couple last week at a country club. The bride and groom interrupted the reception and—tuxedo and flowing gown notwithstanding—went out and played the eighteenth hole.

The list of priests who will be available for reassignment this year has just been issued. There are twenty-five names on it.

"I took a look and crossed off seven right away and then the young curate over at Immaculate Conception went through it for me and penciled out even more," Father Greer says. "He knows the younger bunch. That left eight of them, eight worth talking about. And they have to contact us. I haven't heard of anybody beating down the doors here; no calls. So when our young Father Rossi leaves, those shoes aren't going to be filled. If the folks have been grumbling, wait till they see the new Mass schedule we'll have to put in."

Monsignor Mahoney noisily chews at his last bite of roast beef, his response a mixture of a snort and a chortle as it emerges filtered through a half-filled mouth.

Father Greer rests his head in his hands, his arms straddling the empty plate before him. His eyes are bloodshot, yet somehow clear. He shakes his head slowly from side to side.

"As they say, if you don't laugh, you . . ."

His face breaks into a tired grin. He looks up, confronted by a huge piece of lemon meringue pie.

"Father?" says Jessica Williams, who helps in the kitchen at the evening meal. "Are you through yet?"

And who, after reading this miserable journal, every line of which reveals my weakness, my wretched weakness, who would not understand? Is this the showing of a leader, the head of a parish, a guardian of souls?

AFTERWORD

After his return to St. Patrick's in April, Father Greer began to spend most weekends at the rectory. By summer, claiming "It's better to be here all week than to try to do a week's work in a weekend," he moved in, to live there full time and resume his duties as pastor.

His low blood counts persisted, but he was able to extend the period between his visits to the New England Medical Center first to two weeks and eventually to a month. He did not return to Ireland for his aunt's fiftieth anniversary.

Although his strength improved, he continued to experience extreme fatigue, because of the low blood counts. Dr. Desforges administered two experimental drugs to help stimulate cell growth and also gave Father Greer the seven and eighth sacks of his frozen stem cells. His blood counts did not improve.

Father Greer's depression was so pronounced that, late in the fall, Dr. Desforges called him in to her office for a long private talk. She sympathized with him on the burden of the fatigue but told him that, while his counts were low, they were certainly capable of sustaining life, and that there was no reason why he could not and should not live a productive, though somewhat circumscribed, life. There was no sign of the myeloma.

Within a week of this conversation, Father Greer's spirits seemed to lift. And so did his blood counts, holding at the highest levels (near 30 for red cells, 2.4 for white) since the transplant.

Unfortunately, the counts then dropped back to their previous levels.

By December, John Andrews was bedridden with the effects of his myeloma. He feared death, he told Father Greer. Through numerous visits to Andrews before Christmas, the priest prepared his fellow patient for what they both knew was inevitable. On Christmas Eve, Andrews said, "I'm ready now." Father Greer said Mass for Andrews and his family in their home on Christmas Day and buried him a week later.

At about the same time—the end of 1989—some six months after he had returned to St. Patrick's, evidence of multiple myeloma was again found in Father Greer's blood samples. Although troubling, the low-grade presence of the disease was not seen by Father Greer's doctors as requiring immediate treatment.

Father Greer was by then deep into his next project, the renovation of the upper church. Monsignor Mahoney had moved out, to a retirement home, and a seminary classmate, a retired navy chaplain, had moved in to help out. Father Greer continued to say daily Mass, baptize, marry, bury, and generally carry out the functions of the pastor of a large church. He continued to receive periodic transfusions and, because of a buildup of iron in his system—potentially dangerous to his heart and liver functions— each evening he would insert beneath his skin a hypodermic needle that, with the aid of a small pump, would inject a medication that removed excess iron from his body.

In May 1991—some two and a half years after the bone marrow transplant—the disease, although still at a low level, had advanced to a point where Father Greer's doctors at New England Medical Center began radiation therapy and prescribed prednisone, a steroid drug. By the end of July the disease was again in remission.

Near the end of the year, upon returning from a golfing vacation in Georgia, Father Greer experienced extreme fatigue and pain in the area of his ribs where the myeloma had once been lodged. Although he tried to brush off these symptoms, determined to wait until his next scheduled clinic appointment, he finally called Dr. Desforges who, after hearing the symptoms, told him to come as soon as he could. When he arrived a few hours later, Father Greer was sweating profusely and, to Dr. Desforges' trained eye, on the verge of collapse. She immediately had him admitted.

The pneumonia she discovered quickly worsened. Father Greer's immune system, made fragile by both his disease and the many steroids he had been administered, could not fight off the infection. A staph infection raced through Father Greer's body; his temperature soared to 104 degrees. As 90 percent of his lung capacity was impaired, he had great difficulty breathing. He was rushed from Proger 6 to the Medical Intensive Care Unit where he was heavily sedated with morphine before a breathing tube was placed down his throat.

Unconscious, Father Greer lingered between life and death for ten days. Slowly, antibiotics overcame the infection. When he was finally returned to Proger 6, he could not remember being admitted to the hospital. After a month in the hospital, he was sent to the Spaulding Rehabilitation Hospital in Boston, where he was given intensive physical therapy. At first, he could take no more than a few steps with the assistance of a walker and a plastic brace on this left leg, which suffered nerve damage. He eventually went to convalesce at Immaculate Conception Church in Everett, where he had lived after the bone marrow transplant. His strength continued to return. His doctors once again found no evidence of myeloma present in his blood samples. Actually, his blood counts were as good as they had even been since the transplant.

Before traveling to Florida to spend February and March 1992 with friends, he wrote a short column for the parish bulletin, under the heading "From the Pastor's Desk." He acknowledged the careful attention he had received at both the medical center and the rehabilitation hospital. He continued:

"But the ones I am totally indebted to are the members of the community of St. Patrick's: men, women and children who prayed and stormed heaven for my recovery. I believe it was you who made the difference between life and death. I believe that it was only through your prayers that we were able to conquer this illness. . . . It is with great pride that I boast that I am the pastor of St. Patrick's Church, Natick; a parish that ranks second to none. . . . God Bless, Fr. Greer."

Father Greer planned to return on Palm Sunday, April 12, 1992, and once again take up his responsibilities—"with God's help," as he would say—as pastor of his church.

PAUL WILKES
Hardwick, Massachusetts
March 1, 1992

About the Author

In addition to his books, PAUL WILKES has written for many magazines, including *The New Yorker, The New York Times Magazine,* and *The Atlantic.* He has produced, directed, written, or hosted documentaries for public television, including the series *Six American Families* and *Merton,* a film biography of Thomas Merton. He has been the visiting writer at Clark University, the University of Pittsburgh, and other schools. He lives with his wife, Tracy, and sons, Noah and Daniel, in Hardwick, Massachusetts.